GENETICS AND GENOMICS
FOR THE CARDIOLOGIST

BASIC SCIENCE FOR THE CARDIOLOGIST

1. B. Swynghedauw (ed.): *Molecular Cardiology for the Cardiologist.* Second Edition. 1998   ISBN 0-7923-8323-0

2. B. Levy, A. Tedgui (eds.): *Biology of the Arterial Wall.* 1999
                                                        ISBN 0-7923-8458-X

3. M.R. Sanders, J.B. Kostis (eds.): *Molecular Cardiology in Clinical Practice.* 1999   ISBN 0-7923-8602-7

4. B.Ostadal, F. Kolar (eds.): *Cardiac Ischemia: From Injury to Protection.* 1999
                                                        ISBN 0-7923-8642-6

5. H. Schunkert, G.A.J. Riegger (eds.): *Apoptosis in Cardiac Biology.* 1999
                                                        ISBN 0-7923-8648-5

6. A. Malliani, (ed.): *Principles of Cardiovascular Neural Regulation in Health and Disease.* 2000   ISBN 0-7923-7775-3

7. P. Benlian: *Genetics of Dyslipidemia.* 2001   ISBN 0-7923-7362-6

8. D. Young: *Role of Potassium in Preventive Cardiovascular Medicine.* 2001
                                                        ISBN 0-7923-7376-6

9. E. Carmeliet, J. Vereecke: *Cardiac Cellular Electrophysiology.* 2002
                                                        ISBN 0-7923-7544-0

10. C. Holubarsch: *Mechanics and Energetics of the Myocardium.* 2002
                                                        ISBN 0-7923-7570-X

11. J.S. Ingwall: *ATP and the Heart.* 2002   ISBN 1-4020-7093-4

12. W.C. De Mello, M.J. Janse: *Heart Cell Coupling and Impuse Propagation in Health and Disease.* 2002   ISBN 1-4020-7182-5

13. P.P.-Dimitrow: *Coronary Flow Reserve – Measurement and Application: Focus on transthoracic Doppler echocardiography.* 2002   ISBN 1-4020-7213-9

14. G.A. Danieli: *Genetics and Genomics for the Cardiologist.* 2002
                                                        ISBN 1-4020-7309-7

KLUWER ACADEMIC PUBLISHERS – DORDRECHT/BOSTON/LONDON

GENETICS AND GENOMICS FOR THE CARDIOLOGIST

Gian Antonio Danieli

Professor of Human Genetics

University of Padua

Distributors for North, Central and South America:
Kluwer Academic Publishers
101 Philip Drive
Assinippi Park
Norwell, Massachusetts 02061 USA
Telephone (781) 871-6600
Fax (781) 681-9045
E-Mail: kluwer@wkap.com

Distributors for all other countries:
Kluwer Academic Publishers Group
Post Office Box 322
3300 AH Dordrecht, THE NETHERLANDS
Telephone 31 786 576 000
Fax 31 786 576 254
E-Mail: services@wkap.nl

 Electronic Services <http://www.wkap.nl>

Library of Congress Cataloging-in-Publication Data

Danieli, Gian Antonio, 1942-
   Genetics and genomics for the cardiologist / Gian Antonio Danieli.
     p. ; cm. -- (Basic science for the cardiologist ; 14)
   Includes bibliographical references and index.
   ISBN 1-4020-7309-7 (hbk. : alk. paper)
    1. Congenital heart disease--Genetic aspects. 2. Medical genetics. 3. Human genetics.
4. Genomics. I. Title. II. Series.
    [DNLM: 1. Cardiovascular Abnormalities--genetics. 2. Cardiovascular
Diseases--genetics. 3. Genetic Screening--methods. 4. Genetics, Biochemical. WG 220
D184g 2002]
   RC687 D365 2002
   616.1'042--dc21

                                           2002035294

CONTENTS

PREFACE

In the last twenty years, we have witnessed unprecedented progress in human and medical genetics. The most evident and outstanding result was the release of the nearly completed sequence of the entire human genome into the public domain in February 2001. This was the triumph of the "reverse genetics revolution" started in early 70's. One year later, almost all genes in the human genome are identified, although the function of the encoded products is still unknown for many of them.

The application of molecular genetics to the study of human disease has enabled researchers to discover the majority of genes whose mutations cause diseases inherited as Mendelian traits, however, the identification of genes involved in "common" diseases, such as coronary atherosclerosis has just begun.

The relevance of molecular genetics to medicine is generally acknowledged, but most physicians are still unaware of potential changes in clinical practice as a consequence of recent developments of molecular genetics.

Research on the human genome and other genomes (from viruses, bacteria and yeast to invertebrates and vertebrates) is quickly progressing and fuelling the very rapid development of the novel discipline, genomics, which, in turn, is fuelling the development of proteomics and metabolomics. We are living in a fascinating scientific age, in which knowledge develops at incredible speed.

A person who received his degree in medicine ten years ago may encounter some difficulties when reading genetically oriented papers, unless he or she has continuously refreshed their knowledge in the field. In addition, medical students are often overwhelmed by the details of present discoveries of human molecular genetics.

I recently read the following quote in an authoritative cardiology journal: "It is easy to become mesmerised by advances in Genetics." Without a full understanding of the basic principles of genetics and genomics, it is difficult to judge the relevance, at present and in perspective, of novel diagnostics and therapeutics, derived from these advancements.

The aim of this book is to provide updated and concise information on recent developments in these fields, with particular reference to cardiology. I was forced to omit two important topics, such as immunogenetics and population genetics as writing about them in some detail would have exceedingly increased the size of this volume.

I selected to skip "classical" Genetics and instead to introduce in the first chapter, the "old" Genetics into the new conceptual frame of Genomics.

The second chapter details the relationships between genome and clinical phenotype. Chapter three focuses on methods for identification of disease genes in humans. A section of this chapter is dedicated to multifactorial diseases which are presently the focus of both genetic and medical research.

Chapter 4 is dedicated to inherited structural and functional defects of the myocardium. In this field, relevant progress has been made in recent years. Several involved genes were identified, pathogenic mutations were detected and described and, in some cases, genotype-phenotype correlations were established.

Chapter 5 is dedicated to inherited cardiovascular disorders, with particular reference to coronary atherosclerotic disease and to hypertension.

Finally, Chapter 6 focuses on genetics and genomics applied to diagnosis and therapy, with particular emphasis on recent developments in genetic testing and gene-based therapeutics.

I tried my best to avoid redundancy, focus on facts, and maintain a plain scientific language. I hope that the presence of several explanatory figures, a Glossary, and many references might provide additional help to the Reader.

Three Appendices are included in the text: Appendix I contains a list of websites which contain updated information on genetics and molecular genetics of cardiovascular disorders. Several additional URLs (Internet addresses) are located within the text. Appendix II provides, for each of 128 inherited cardiovascular diseases and genetic disorders with relevant cardiac involvement, the ID number in the OMIM database. In Appendix III, known genes encoding ionic channels and expressed in the human heart are listed.

I hope this volume will succeed to enable the reader to master a subject that is already part of clinical practice, but will no doubt become more and more important for the cardiologist in the near future.

Padua, June 28, 2002

Acknowledgements

I would like to thank first Professor B. Swynghedauw, who suggested me to write this book.

Several persons kindly accepted to be the alfa-test of my writing and contributed to the final version with their helpful criticisms: Dr. A. Bagattin, Dr. G. Beffagna, Dr. A. Bisognin, Dr. S. Bortoluzzi, Dr. G. Lanfranchi, Dr. A. Rampazzo, Dr. P. Melacini, Dr. C. Veronese. and Dr. L. Vitiello. I am very grateful to them all.

Most artwork is due to the skill of Mr. R. Mazzaro, to whom I am particularly indebted for his unvaluable help. Mrs. Karen Gustafson kindly revised the English.

Last, but not least, I wish to thank my wife Luisella, for her full understanding and support.

G.A.D.

CHAPTER 1

THE HUMAN GENOME

1.1 Size and characteristics of nuclear and mitochondrial genome in humans

The total genetic complement of our species is called "human genome". It comprises a set of different DNA molecules, corresponding to 25 different types of chromosomes (22 autosomes, X chromosome, Y chromosome, mitochondrial DNA) which are present within our cells. All these DNA molecules are transmitted from cell to cell and from generation to generation: chromosomes by mitosis and meiosis, mitochondrial DNA by replication followed by mitochondrial fission and by random inclusion in the cytoplasm of daughter cells after cell cleavage. Since mitochondria of the zygote are almost exclusively contributed by the cytoplasm of the female gamete, genes carried by mitochondrial DNA (mtDNA) follow the rules of "maternal inheritance" or "cytoplasmic inheritance". In principle, mutations in mitochondrial DNA will be transmitted to all the children of the same mother, but only daughters will pass a mtDNA mutation to next generation. On the contrary, mutations in DNA carried by chromosomes will follow the rules dictated by chromosomal duplication, recombination and segregation.

A "gene" corresponds to a segment of DNA which could be transcribed into an RNA molecule (which, according to the cases, may be mRNA, rRNA or tRNA). In case of protein-coding genes, transcript (mRNA) is then translated into a polypeptide. Each gene occupies a definite place along the chromosomal DNA. By convention, location of each gene on the DNA molecule is expressed as a distance from a given reference point: the short arm telomere in each chromosome and the origin of replication in the mitochondrial DNA. Both the length of a segment of DNA and its distance from the reference point are measured in nucleotide units: Kb (1 kilobase = 1,000 nucleotides) and Mb (1 megabase = 1,000,000 nucleotides).

A draft of the DNA sequence of each human chromosome is now available on-line, on public domain, at the website Human Genome Browser, at the University of California,Santa Cruz (http://genome.ucsc.edu/) , or at the website of the European Bioinformatic Institute (http://ensemble.ebi.ac.uk/). Each chromosome is represented there as a virtual line, on which genes and DNA markers are placed at proper distance one from another. A powerful browser enables to locate the wanted segment by typing its name (e.g. the name of a given gene or the ID of a given DNA marker) or simply by typing in an appropriate box the nucleotide sequence corresponding to the wanted segment or to part of it.

Length in Mb of all human chromosomes (22 autosomes, plus the sex chromosomes X and Y) and of human mitochondrial DNA is reported in Tab 1.1.

Table 1.1: Length of different chromosomes of the human genome, expressed in megabases (Mb) of DNA.

Cromosome	Mb	Cromosome	Mb
1	263	13	114
2	255	14	109
3	214	15	106
4	203	16	98
5	194	17	92
6	183	18	85
7	171	19	67
8	155	20	72
9	145	21	50
10	144	22	56
11	144	X	164
12	143	Y	59
		Mt DNA	0.0166

If we compare the length of mitochondrial DNA (16.6 kb) with the total length of DNA molecules corresponding to human chromosomes of the haploid set (over 3,000 Mb), we see that its coding capacity is exceedingly modest (about 0.0005% of the total). Even taking into account that in every diploid human cell we have only two sets of chromosomes but thousands of mitochondrial DNAs, the total mitocondrial contribution to genomic DNA can account for no more than 0.5% of the DNA in a single cell. Nevertheless, mutations affecting genes carried by mitochondrial DNA may be as harmful as those occurring in genes carried by nuclear chromosomes.

As far as the gene content is concerned, mtDNA contains 37 genes, 22 of which encode different mt tRNAs, 2 code for mt rRNAs and 13 encode polypeptides which are subunits of mitochondrial enzymes. The structure and function of mitochondrion is specified by these 13 genes of the mtDNA, plus additional 50 genes, carried by different nuclear chromosomes.

The number of nuclear genes is still unknown but, according to recent estimates, it could be between 35,000 and 60,000.

1.2 Structural and functional organization of human chromosomes

Mitochondrial DNA is a single, double-stranded DNA molecule with very little repetitive DNA. About 95% of mtDNA corresponds to coding sequences. Genes are intronless. They are located on both strands, with a density of 1/0.45 Kb. Transcription of each strand generates large multi-genic mRNA molecules, which are subsequently cleaved.

On the contrary, DNA of each nuclear chromosome is a single, linear and double-stranded molecule, uninterrupted from telomere to telomere (Fig. 1.1).

A metaphase chromosome is made by two linear double-stranded DNA molecules, derived from the previous DNA replication and connected by protein complexes in correspondence of a relatively small region (which position is typical for each chromosome), called "centromere".

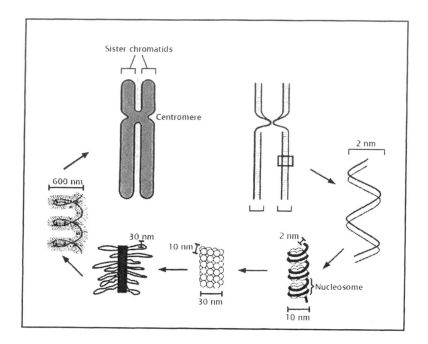

Figure 1.1: A metaphase chromosome corresponds to two double-helices of DNA (chromatids), complexed with nuclear proteins, coiled and supercoiled (from Strachan, modified).

If the DNA of a single human chromosome would be fully uncoiled, a very long molecule would result, ranging in length from a minimum of 1.7 cm (chromosome 22 and chromosome Y) to a maximum of 8.5 cm (chromosome 1). On the contrary, due to coiling and super-coiling, human metaphase chromosomes appear as tiny structures, about 1 micron thick, ranging from 2 to 10 microns in length.

Chromosomal DNA is rich in repetitive sequences, which occur as tandemly repeats, clustered repeats or interspersed repeats. Some tandemly repeated sequences may span some Kb and occur in tens or hundreds of copies. Interspersed repetitive DNA sequences have in general smaller size, but they occur in thousand to million copies. The different types of interspersed repeats probably account in total for over 25% of the whole genomic DNA.

Most genomic DNA (possibly 45%) is made of extragenic DNA, occurring as unique sequences or in low copy number. According to present knowledge, derived from the results of the Human Genome Project, the DNA of a chromosome may be viewed as a very long sequence of nucleotides in which we may identify specific segments, on the basis of their sequence peculiarities (Fig. 1.2).

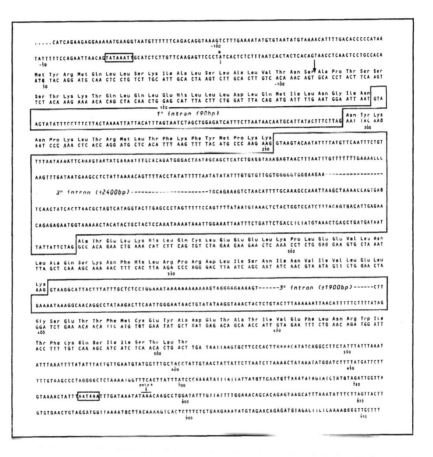

Figure 1.2 : A stretch of DNA sequence from human genome. The sequence of the complementary strand was omitted for simplicity. Software for gene prediction detected the TATA box of the promoter region (little box on the top of the figure) and three exons. The correspondence between codons and aminoacids is shown. Intronic sequences (boxed in the figure) are partially omitted (fom McKonkey, modified).

For instance, the presence of a DNA segment which, because of the nucleotide consensus sequence, could be attributed to a promoter, would indicate that probably there is a gene downstream, in close proximity. Similarly, the absence of stop codons in a relatively long stretch of DNA would identify an ORF (Open Reading Frame), probably corresponding to one exon.

Specific software is now available to researchers for inspecting genomic DNA sequences, in order to quickly identify possible genes and their regulatory sequences.

Presently, genes identified by bioinformatic search on genomic DNA sequences ("predicted" genes) are exceedingly more numerous than those identified by traditional cloning methods. Many of them are still waiting for functional characterization.

1.3   Structural and functional organization of human genes

Most protein-coding genes have a complex internal organization. A typical gene consists in a primary regulatory region ("promoter"), in two untranslated regions (5' UTR and 3' UTR) and in a series of coding segments ("exons"), separated by other segments, which are transcribed, but not translated ("introns") (Fig. 1.3).

Before being associated with ribosomes and translated into a polypeptide, the product of transcription (primary transcript) is processed, by removal of intronic sequences ("splicing").

In very large genes, the process of transcription and subsequent splicing may require several hours. It has been calculated that over 10 hours would be required to a cardiomyocyte to transcribe a gene coding for dystrophin or for ryanodine receptor protein.

Through inclusion or exclusion of specific exons from the processed transcript (alternative splicing), a single gene may produce different protein products (Fig. 1.4).

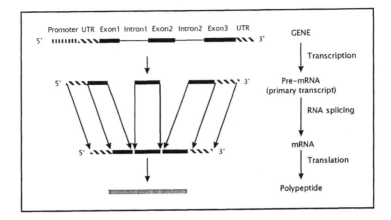

Figure 1.3: Sketch of the process of gene expression. The primary transcript undergoes splicing before being translated into a polypeptide.

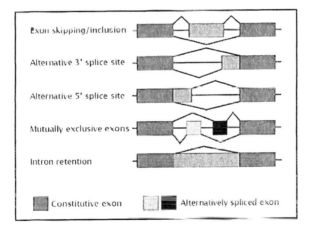

Figure 1.4: Different possibilities of alternative splicing. (from Modrek, modified)

Size of human genes is very variable, from very small (e.g. Histone H4: 0.4 Kb; alpha-interferon: 0.9 Kb) to giant genes (e.g. dystrophin: 2,300 Kb). In general, larger is the gene, higher is the number of its exons and higher is the proportion of its intronic DNA (up to 99%).

In the whole, coding DNA sequences account for a small fraction of the total genomic DNA, possibly 3%. However, since the large majority of genes include introns, the portion of genomic DNA really occupied by genes is probably much larger. For instance, exons of the human gene coding for the cardiac ryanodine receptor (hRyR2) account in total for about 15 kb, but the whole gene, including introns and regulatory sequences, spans over 1.5 Mb.

Often genes occur in clusters, separated by stretches of non-coding extragenic DNA. Within these clusters not infrequently genes occur on both strands, in opposite direction. Not infrequently, coding sequences laying on one strand correspond to part of intronic sequences of the opposite strand (Fig.1.5).

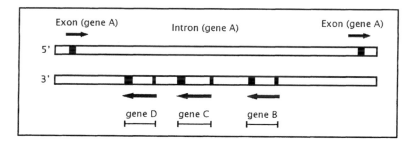

Figure 1.5: Genes are carried on both strands of DNA. Sometime, like in this figure, small genes may correspond to an intronic sequence on the opposite strand (from Strachan, modified).

In the past, the small proportion of coding sequences compared with that of extragenic DNA in the human genome suggested that clusters of genes could be separated by very long sequences of non-coding DNA. This view is presently challenged by the observation that many human genes span a long

DNA sequence, in spite of the relatively short total length of coding sequences.

Probably, most of genomic human DNA is occupied by genes, if we consider their coding and non-coding segments. However, different concentration of genes in different chromosomes and in different regions of the same chromosome is probable.

In human genome there are also non-functional copies of genes, called "pseudogenes". Although their DNA sequence is closely similar to that of functional genes, they are inactive because of deletions, insertions or stop codons, or mutations in regulatory sequences. They probably derive from gene duplications and often they lay closely to their functional counterparts. A different and peculiar class of pseudogenes ("processed pseudogenes"), correspond to products of reverse transcription (DNA produced on an RNA template), subsequently integrated in the chromosomal DNA, at random, as shown in Fig. 1.6.

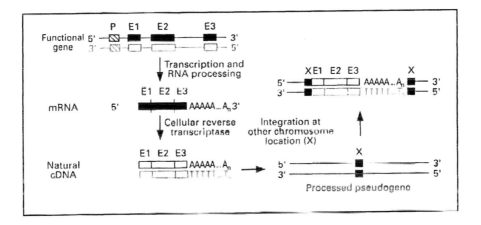

Figure 1.6 : Generation of a processed pseudogene
(from Strachan, modified)

Processed preudogenes are functionally inactive, but in human genome there are tens of fully functional intronless genes, which are believed to derive from events of reverse transcription, followed by chromosomal integration.

1.4 Artificial banding of human chromosomes

Each human chromosome is a very long stretch of double stranded DNA, along which we encounter genes and clusters of genes, interspersed in repetitive or highly repetitive DNA sequences.

During interphase, the period of the cell cycle in which cells are involved in their differentiated activity, chromosomes are mostly de-condensed, although some regions (heterocromatic regions) remain compacted. De-condensed chromosomal structure is available to the process of transcription of genes.

At the pro-metaphase of the mitosis or meiosis, chromosomes undergo a progressive compaction, until they appear at the metaphase as condensed structures. When gently de-proteinized and stained with Giemsa, human metaphase chromosomes reveal a banding pattern, typical for each chromosome (Fig. 1.7).

Each band corresponds, in average, to about 6 Mb of DNA. In dark bands (G-bands) DNA is tightly packed, while in negatively staining bands ("interbands") chromosomal structure is more relaxed. According to its banding pattern, each chromosome was subdivided into regions and sub-regions.

A convention adopted since 1970, enabled to establish cytogenetic maps for each chromosome. A simple notation enables to refer unambiguously to each specific chromosomal segment: after the number indicating the chromosome, p means short arm, q long arm, the first number the region, the second number the sub-region (band) and the third one the sub-subregion.

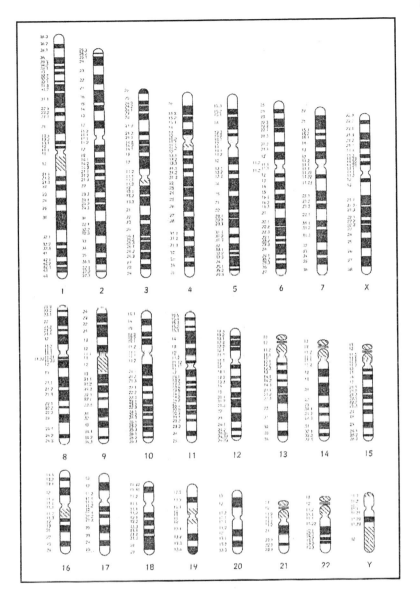

Figure 1.7: Standard Giemsa staining (450 G-bands). Chromatids of each chromosome are not shown.(from Strachan, modified)

About 450 different bands can be detected in a standard metaphase preparation, while high-resolution banding (performed on pro-metaphase chromosomes) reveals about 800 bands.

This method is routinely used to screen chromosomes for alterations in number or structure, in case of malformations or suspected cytogenetic abnormalities in patients.

1.5 Replication of human DNA and the origin of new mutations

Every cell division is preceded by DNA replication. During this process, in different points along the double-stranded DNA molecule, helicase unwinds the DNA duplex and the two complementary strands are copied to daughter complementary molecules by DNA polymerase. Since each of two daughter double-stranded DNA molecules is made by one parental single-strand and by its complementary copy, this process is called "semi-conservative" replication. At the end, the entire chromosomal DNA will be copied in two identical and double stranded DNA molecules. Each chromosome will result longitudinally subdivided into two sister chromatids, each containing a long double-stranded DNA molecule.

The two double-stranded DNA molecules originated by replication are virtually identical, but several errors may intervene during DNA replication and many substitutions, deletions or additions of nucleotides may occur. In spite of efficient systems of DNA repair, at every DNA replication several variations are introduced in novel DNA sequences.

It has been estimated that for a DNA segment spanning about 2 Kb, the rate of spontaneous error (spontaneous mutation rate) is about 1/ 10,000,000 (1 mutant over 10,000,000 copies) per cell division. However, what is commonly referred as "mutation rate" in humans is much higher (probably over 1/1,000,000 per cell generation), since it includes the mutagenic effect of a variety of chemicals and radiations in nature. If we accept the current estimate of about 40,000 human genes, in every generation, about 4% of gametes would expectedly carry one novel mutation in one of our genes.

If in a single individual, selected at random in human population, a stretch of DNA sequence of one individual chromosome would be compared with its homologue, certainly several differences in the nucleotide sequence would be detected. This rather surprising variability is produced by spontaneous mutation occurring in every generation. Only a fraction of such variability is relevant to human health, restricted to pathogenic mutations in some genes.

1.6 Effects of mutations in DNA sequences

Mutations involving a single nucleotide or a small number of nucleotides are called "micro-lesions" or "point" mutations. They are mostly generated by errors occurring during DNA replication.

In the most simple case, i.e. a single-nucleotide substitution, different consequences are possible. Due to the degeneracy of the genetic code (different codons specify the same aminoacid) the substitution might produce no apparent change ("silent" or "synonymous" or "neutral" mutation). Alternatively, a non-synonymous mutation might result, due to the origin of a novel codon, specifying a different aminoacid. Synonymous and non-synonymous mutations are often referred as "missense" mutations.

In case of a non-synonymous mutation, the aminoacid change might be radical (e.g. from non-polar to polar) or mild (e.g. from one polar to another polar aminoacid). The functional consequences of such changes would depend not only on the kind of aminoacidic substitution, but also on the site where it occurred within the molecule. Often, critical sites (e.g. phosphorylation sites) are very vulnerable and even mild modifications in their aminoacid sequence may produce relevant functional changes.

A single-nucleotide substitution may also produce a stop codon ("nonsense" mutation). In this case a "truncated" protein will result, frequently inactive and prematurely degraded within the cell.

Addition or deletion of 3 nucleotides or of a number of nucleotides multiple of 3 would maintain the correct reading frame in the DNA sequence.

In all alternative cases, the reading frame will be lost. As a consequence, in the sequence downstream the deletion (or the insertion) a stop codon would be generated by chance in the novel frame of reading and the translation into protein will be prematurely terminated ("frameshift" mutations).

In the case of an in-frame deletion, the resulting polypeptide would lack of one or more aminoacids, leading to possible functional alterations, especially when the deletion involves a functionally relevant region of the protein.

An in-frame insertion would introduce a certain number of novel codons, among which one might be, by chance, a stop codon ("nonsense" mutation). Even neglecting this possibility, addition of novel aminoacids in a polypeptide may lead to alterations in its functional properties, in particular when a functionally relevant domain of the molecule undergoes a significant distortion.

In general, we may say that frame-shift mutations and nonsense mutations are deleterious, while missense mutation are not always pathogenic.

Mutations (nucleotide substitutions, deletions or insertions) may occur also within splicing consensus sequences (splicing acceptors and donors). The alteration of one of such sequences usually induces exon skipping, with consequent deletion of part of the transcript. In some cases, the situation may be worsened by the joining of two ends which do not necessarily have a precise correspondence of reading frame.

Let's assume that exon 1 ends with the third letter of the last codon, while exon 2 ends with the second letter of its last codon. In case of skipping of exon 2, the first exon would still remain in frame and would still end with the third letter of its last codon. However, reading frame would continue in exon 3 with the third letter of a codon. Therefore, a downstream frame-shift would be generated by abnormal junction between exon1 and exon3.

Point mutations may also occur within introns: in this case they may convert a "cryptic" splicing site (i.e. a short DNA sequence mimicking a splicing consensus sequence) into an active splicing site.

The resulting novel splicing pattern might grossly modify the transcript; it even might introduce in the novel trancript a segment of intronic sequence containing a stop codon, thus producing the arrest of translation.

Although mutations occur at random, characteristics of the DNA sequence (the so-called "DNA sequence environment") may increase the probability of mutation in given nucleotides or in limited segments of DNA. For this reason, in some genes mutational "hot-spots" may be encountered.

A brief summary of types of typical "point" mutations and of their effects is shown in Tab. 1.2.

Table 1.2: Types of "point" mutations

TYPE OF MUTATION	EFFECTS	
Synonymous	No change in aminoacid	
Missense	Change in aminoacid	
	-	with similar properties
	-	with different properties
Nonsense	Generation of a stop codon	
Frame–shift	Alteration of the reading frame	
Splicing–site	Modification of the splicing site	

A different type of mutation is the so-called "triplet repeat expansion". This kind of mutation has been reported so far in a limited number of human genes, as typical pathogenic variation. These genes normally include a variable number of triplet repeats (CAG, CTG, CGG, GAA, CCG or GCC). In some genes the repeats are in the coding region, in others in one of the UTRs, in others in the promoter. The number of repeats may undergo abnormal amplification, thus leading to gene dysfunction.

A typical case of disease due to triplet repeat expansion is myotonic dystrophy (Steinert's disease), a neuromuscular disorder in which cardiological symptoms (conduction defects, mitral valve prolapse and wall motion defects) are frequently observed.

Normally, gene DMPK (Dystrophia Myotonica Protein Kinase) shows, at its 3' UTR, from 5 to 30 copies of CTG. In individuals afftected with a mild form of Steinert Disease, from 50 to 80 copies may be detected instead, while in severely affected individuals more than 2,000 copies may be found.

High number of triplets (expansion) is pathogenic, possibly related to alteration of splicing in the region close to 3' UTR of the DMPK gene. Number of repeats correlate with severity of the affection.

In theory, the number of repeats should be regularly inherited from generation to generation. On the contrary, while small numbers of repeats (from 5 to 18) are inherited according to this rule, larger numbers of repeats (from 19 to 37) demonstrate to be "unstable" and prone to increase, possibly because DNA polymerase slippage. Individuals carrying over 50 repeats are still fully asymptomatic, but this number of repeats is highly unstable and it is considered a state of "pre-mutation". Futher increase in number of repeats is possibly due to frequent unequal crossing-over, or to unequal sister-chromatid exchange. The same processes may eventually produce a decrease in number of triplets; for this reason, pathogenic mutations due to triplet repeat expansion are called "dynamic mutations".

It is interesting to notice that instability may induce large variability in number of repeats also in different tissues of the same individual, thus leading to variability in clinical presentation. Moreover, number of repeats detected in lymphocyte DNA may be different from that which could be detected in skeletal muscle or in myocardial cells.

In some cases, genetic disease may be due to modifications involving large or very large stretches of DNA, which may include part of a gene, an entire gene or several genes.

This kind of mutation may be considered as chromosomal structural alterations and/or rearrangements. They include deletions and duplications of chromosomal segments, or deletions followed by translocation in a different place or in a different chromosome. The involved DNA sequences are variable in length (from less than 1 Kb to several Mb). When size is in the range of megabases, the alteration may be detected also at cytogenetic level as "chromosomal structural aberration".

Pathogenic effect of such mutations may arise from gross alterations in a single gene (e.g. partial deletion of the coding sequence of a gene involved in a translocation) or in several genes (e.g. deletions of several contiguous gene = contiguous gene deletion syndrome in males showing a micro-deletion of the X chromosome). If DNA segment involved in the structural aberration is very large, pathogenic effect may arise from unbalanced dosage in several genes (see Chapter 2, section 2.7). Table 1.3 summarizes the effects of different types of mutations.

Table 1.3: Possible effects of different types of mutations

TYPE	EFFECTS
Extragenic mutation	May inactivate regulatory elements
Promoter mutation	Altered expression.
Promoter deletion	Abolishes transcription
Exonic mutation	May produce a stop codon or an aminoacid change
Splice site mutation	May induce exon skipping or intron retention
Intronic mutations	May activate cryptic splicing sites
Termination codon	Additional aminoacids may be included, before a novel stop
Poly(A) signals	Expression may be altered. Deletion abolishes
Exon deletion	Protein domain missing. Often downsream frame–shift
Intron deletion	No effect
Whole gene deletion	No product in hemizygosis. Dosage effect in heterozygosis
Whole gene duplication	Possible dosage effect
Multigene deletion	In hemizygosis contiguous gene syndrome. Dosage effects
Multigene duplication	Dosage effects

According to statistics on 25,256 mutations in 1,132 human genes, micro-lesions (i.e. "point" mutations) would account for over 90% of the total; missense and nonsense mutations would be the most frequent alteration in absolute terms. (Tab.1.4). However, frequency of mutations causing exon-skipping are probably underestimated, since they can be detected only through

18

the analysis of cDNA obtained from a tissue specimen, a procedure which is seldom applied when looking for mutations in a given gene.

Table 1.4: Statistics of different types of mutations detected in human genes (from Human Gene Mutation Database, Feb.2002)

Micro-lesions		*93.07*
Missense/nonsense	4,966	59.25
Splicing	2,501	9.90
Regulatory	190	0.75
Small deletions	4,149	16.43
Small insertions	1,536	6.08
Small ins/del	172	0.68
Gross lesions		*6.91*
Repeat expansions	34	0.13
Insertions/duplications	151	0.60
Complex rearrangements	276	1.11
Gross deletions	1,281	5.07
TOTAL	*25,256*	*100.00*

1.7 DNA markers

When occurring in extra-genic non-coding DNA, mutations do not produce effects in terms of proteins, and have no effect on the clinical phenotype. In theory, a deletion of several Kb of extra-genic DNA could be harmless.

Like mutations in coding sequences, mutations in non-coding DNA, once originated, are transmitted generation after generation. In theory, we should be able to recognize among chromosomes of different individuals a single chromosome in which a given mutation occurred several generations ago. This is really possible, by analyzing human DNA by automatic DNA sequencing or by ancillary techniques like PCR and dHPLC (see Chapter 3).

One mutation in a DNA sequence is like a "label". Therefore, a short sequence of DNA which would include a known mutation may be considered a " DNA marker".

Single-nucleotide substitutions in non-coding DNA and neutral single-nucleotide substitutions in coding DNA are called SNPs (Single Nucleotide Polymorphisms). A DNA variant is considered part of a genetic polymorphism when its frequency in the population is above 0.99% . In the human genome a SNP is encountered approximately every 100-300 nucleotides. At the beginning of 2002, the SNP public database (http://snp.cshl.org/db/map/snp) included over 1.4 million SNPs, all of wich anchored to the human genome sequence working draft.

SNPs are very good DNA markers, which are presently used for mapping genes involved in multifactorial diseases (see Chapter 3) and for attempting to reconstruct the biological history of human populations.

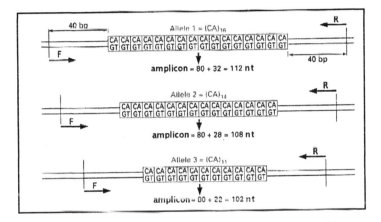

Figure 1.8. Polymorphism of length of PCR amplified products. Amplicons obtained using the two PCR primers F and R, will differ in length, because of the variable number of dinucleotide (CA) repeats within the DNA sequence recognized by the two PCR primers (from Strachan, modified).

A different kind of DNA markers are the so-called "microsatellite markers", corresponding to relatively short DNA sequences including a variable number of dinucleotide repeats. These variable segments of DNA, also named STRPs (Short Tandem Repeat Polymorphisms), are very abundant along every human chromosome; they show a good level of polymorphism (i.e. variability among individuals of the same population) and of heterozygosity (i.e. the probability that a given individual, selected at random

20

in the population, is heterozygous at the selected locus). Microsatellite variants may be easily detected by PCR followed by gel electrophoresis (Fig. 1.8).

Each amplicon corresponds to an individual double-stranded DNA, i.e. to a single homologue. For this reason, mobility variants are "allelic variants" and will segregate as mendelian characters. These allelic variants (or, more simply, "alleles") are classified according to the electrophoretic mobility of the corresponding amplicons. In general, the most slow-moving bands are indicated as corresponding to "allele 1", while other bands are indicated by progressively increasing numbers, according to their increasing electrophoretic mobility.

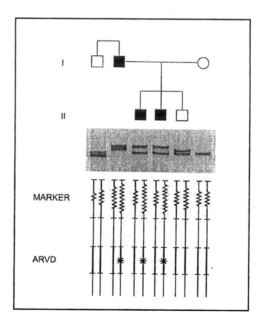

Figure 1.9: At the center of the figure, electrophoretic separation of PCR amplicons obtained from DNAs of different individuals of the family shown on top. Since the marker is closely associated to a disease gene (in this case ARVD), the transmission of the pathogenic allele of such gene (marked by *) can be followed in the family simply by electrophoresis of PCR products. Double bands denote heterozygosity, single bands homozygosity. Electrophoretic mobility of each band depends on number of repeats, indicated by zigzags in the lower part of the figure (see text for details).

An individual showing a single electrophoretic band, will be homozygous or emizygous for the corresponding allele. On the contrary, an individual showing two bands will be heterozygous for the two alleles, identified by the electrophoretic mobility of the corresponding amplicons. For instance, the amplicon 112nt long in Fig.1.8 would correspond to allele 1 and the amplicon 102nt long to allele 3.

By examining results of PCR amplification and of subsequent electrophoretic separation, it is possible to establish which alleles are carried by each single subject (i.e. the "genotype" of the individual for the selected marker), as shown in Fig. 1.9.

In the example reported in Fig. 1.9, mother appears homozygous for a fast-moving band (homozygote for allele 3).

All her sons inherited such a band; two of them inherited from their father, together with the disease, a slow-moving band (allele 1), which is absent in the paternal uncle.

The other son, unaffected, inherited from his father the band with intermediate mobility. Paternal uncle shows one fast-moving band (allele 3) and a "very-fast" band (allele 4), which are not present in his brother. He will be defined as heterozygote 3,4. One of his parents could have been heterozygote 2,3 and the other heterozygote 1,4, but information is insufficient to clarify this point.

The example clearly shows that polymorphic DNA markers may be used for a series of purposes, from paternity testing to linkage studies in families with inherited disorders.

1.8 Chromosomal basis of Inheritance

No matter if a mutation is pathogenic or not, it will be regularly transmitted in cellular generations, by replication and subsequent segregation of the homologue chromosomes at each mitosis (Fig. 1.10). Thus, all somatic cells and germinal cells derived from a zygote carrying a mutation, will carry the same mutation, unless exceptional events would occur. It is interesting to notice that a novel mutation or a chromosomal re-arrangement which would arise in a somatic cell, could originate a cell lineage carrying the mutated DNA sequence. Therefore, there will be a "somatic mosaicism", i.e. the co-existence, within the same individual, of genetically different cell lineages.

If this phenomenon would occur at the time of the multiplication of spermatogones or of the oogones, "gonadal mosaicism" would result.

Because of gonadal mosaicism, a person with apparently normal alleles, may have two children showing the same dominant mutation. While the probability of two independent mutations is extremely low, the possibility of gonadal mosaicism must be seriously taken into consideration in risk assessment.

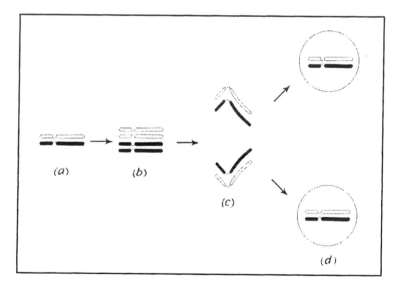

Figure 1.10: Mitosis. Two homologues (a) replicate their DNA during interphase. At metaphase, each chromosome is composed of two sister chromatids. Longitudinal splitting of centromeres and the attachment of each chromatid to the spindle fibers lead to the segregation of two equal chromosomal complements in the two daughter cells.

If the chromosome in white carries a mutation in a gene, this mutation will be transmitted to both daughter cells (for simplicity, only a single pair of homologues is shown).

While normally all cells derived by mitosis would have the same genetic constitution, not all gametes produced by the individual derived from such zygote will be genetically equivalent, because of meiotic segregation of chromosomes (Fig. 1.11).

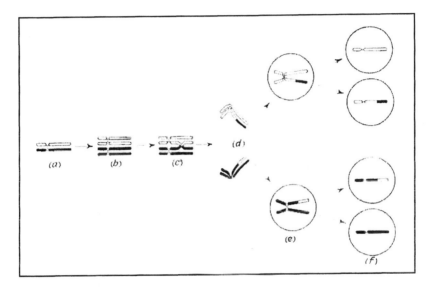

Figure 1.11: Segregation of chromosomes at meiosis. At the prophase of the first meiotic division, recombination (crossing-over) occurs between chromatids of paired homologous chromosomes (c). Recombined chromosomes segregate in the two daughter cells (e). Then, during the second meiotic division, without any further DNA duplication segregation of chromatids occurs (f). In the figure, if the chromosome in white would carry a mutant allele on the tip of its long arm, this mutation would be transmitted to cells inheriting the parental non-recombined white chromosome (1/4 of the total) and in cells which inherited a recombinant chromosome including the tip of the white chromosome. (for simplicity, only one pair of homologues is shown in the figure)

When one zygote receives two copies of the same mutation, one from the male, the other from the female gamete, it is called "homozygote", because they have two identical alleles.

If parents are both heterozygotes for the same mutation, they will have 0.25 (0.5 x 0.5) chance of producing a homozygote. On the other hand, an individual homozygote for a given mutation will produce 100% gametes carrying such variant.

A homozygote may have received one copy of the mutation from the heterozygote parent and the other copy as a new mutation ("fresh" mutation) which occurred in the parent homozygous for normal allele. This situation is, however, relatively infrequent, since mutation is a rare event. A "fresh" mutation may be different from the mutation originally running in the family: it may involve a different nucleotide, or it may be of a different type.

Mutations travel from generation to generation carried by a chromosome, since they are variants of its DNA sequence. They may be transferred to the homologous chromosome by meiotic recombination: in this case there will be a reciprocal exchange of corresponding DNA sequences between the two homologues, mediated by crossing-over .

At metaphase of first meiotic division, homologous chromosomes, each composed of its two chromatids, are pulled apart and migrate toward the pole of the cell in which they will be included. Since in each pair the choice of which homologue would enter which daughter cell is independent for the choice in each of the other chromosome pairs, there will be 2^{23} (over 8 million) possible combinations of parental cromosomes for each meiotic event. On top of that, if we consider that on average each chromosome undergoes recombination in at least two regions at every meiosis, we may realize that an incredibly vast reshuffling of parental chromosomes and chromosomal material takes place at every meiosis.

We can easily trace back in a family the origin and the transmission of DNA variants (pathogenic or neutral they are) through several generations, simply by following the transmission of the chromosome carrying each given variant. On the contrary, it is impossible to precisely predict for each gene which variant (allele) would be contributed by a given parent to a new zygote. In this case, as it happens in risk calculations for genetic counselling, we must rely only on laws of probability.

1.9 The main reference database for human disease-genes

OMIM database (On-line Mendelian Inheritance in Man, http://www.ncbi.nlm.nih.gov./omim/) is the main reference for human genes involved in disease phenotypes. Presently (May 2002), it includes 13,582 entries, with 10,065 established gene loci (7,889 of which are mapped) and 1,058 phenotype descriptions.

Each OMIM entry has a unique six-digit number whose first digit indicates the mode of inheritance of the gene involved. Numbers starting with 1 refer to diseases with autosomal dominant inheritance (entries created before May 15, 1994); those starting with 2 refer to autosomal recessives (entries created before May 15, 1994). Entries indicated by numbers starting with 3 and 4 refer to diseases inherited respectively as X-linked or Y-linked traits. Numbers starting with 5 refer to diseases showing mitochondrial (mtDNA) inheritance, while those starting with 6 refer to autosomal loci, diseases or phenotypes more recently included in the catalogue (entries created after May 15, 1994). An asterisk (*) before an entry number means that the mode of inheritance of the phenotype is reasonably established. The symbol # before an entry number means that disease phenotype may be caused by mutation in any of two or more genes.

OMIM is a searchable database. By inputing a word or a group of words, a list of OMIM entries may be obtained, in which the selected word is contained in the title of the entry or in the text. For instance, by typing "cardiomyopathy restrictive" a list of 14 different entries is obtained. By clicking on OMIM number of each entry, the corresponding web-pages are downloaded, which may be directly printed.

Each OMIM entry provides a brief description of the selected disease, with summary information on biochemical features, molecular genetics, animal models (when available), a series of key references and direct web links to relevant databases, plus a brief clinical synopsis.

Information resident on OMIM is permanently updated, as specified at the end of text of each entry.

OMIM is the most suitable tool for Physicians, whereas other databases of the human genome are mostly addressed to researchers.

1.10 The Human Mutation Database and the nomenclature for human mutations

HUGO (Human Genome Organization) maintains at the EBI (European Bioinformatics Institute) the website "Variation databases" (http://www2.ebi.ac.uk/mutations/cotton/dblist/dblist.html), which collects and manages information on mutations reported in humans.

The website has different sections which are potentially interesting also for clinicians, as "Locus-Specific Mutation Databases" and Complex Disease Databases", with direct link to specialized databases for many human genetic diseases, and "National & Ethnic Mutation Databases", which provide information on geographical distribution of some mutations.

Since the beginning, huge numbers of reported mutations and their large variability forced to adopt a generally accepted nomenclature (Antonarakis, 1988).

Basically, a mutation may be reported with reference to the polynucleotide sequence in which it occurred, or with reference to its consequence, in terms of aminoacid substitution.

In DNA there are four nucleotides: Adenine (A), Thymine (T), Cytosine (C) and Guanine (G). Each gene has a "starting point", called "initiator ATG codon" , from which transcription starts. The A of the initiator codon is considered +1, the reference point for identifying the position of any single nucleotide in the gene and in its flanking sequences. The nucleotide which immediately precedes A in the sequence is considered –1. Therefore, -75G>T means that nucleotide G (Guanine) in position 75 uptream the initiator codon is replaced by T (Thymine); similarly, 1945 G>A means that a Guanine is replaced by Adenine at position 1945, downstream the initiator codon.

Deletions are indicated by writing the two positions coinciding with the edges of the deletion, followed by symbol "del": 5432-5740del means that a deletion occurred including nucleotides from 5432 to 5470. If deletion is limited in size and it is relevant to specify the deleted sequence, the following mode may be used: 3745-3750ATGGA means that deletion of the sequence ATGGAG occurred, starting with nucleotide 3745 and ending with nucleotide 3750.

Table 1.5 : Codes used for indicating single aminoacids in nomenclature for mutations.

A	Alanine	Al
C	Cysteine	Cys
D	Aspartic acid	Asp
E	Glutamic acid	Glu
F	Phenylalanine	Phe
G	Glycine	Gly
H	Histidine	His
I	Isoleucine	Ile
K	Lysine	Lys
M	Methionine	Met
N	Asparagine	Asn
P	Proline	Pro
Q	Glutamine	Gln
R	Arginine	Arg
S	Serine	Ser
T	Threonine	Thr
V	Valine	Val
W	Tryptophane	Try
Y	Tyrosine	Tyr
X	Stop codon	STOP

In case of insertions, the same writing is used, with the only difference that positional data are followed by <u>ins,</u> rather than by <u>del</u>.

When it is important to indicate the consequence of a mutation in terms of aminoacid sequence, rather than the kind of nucleotide substitution, aminoacid codes (Tab. 1.5) are used, instead of nucleotide symbols. In this case the initiator codon is considered as number 1. Therefore, Y210X means that codon 210 specifying Tyrosin, was changed into a stop codon; similarly, S121R means that codon 121, originally specifying Serine, underwent mutation and now specifies Arginine.

The three-letter code for aminoacids, currently used in biochemistry, is also accepted (e.g. Ser121Arg, Tyr210stop). Frequently, a simplified version of the mutation notation is used in scientific reports dealing with variants relevant to human diseases: e.g. "174M" means variation in codon 174, corresponding to a methionine in place of the original aminoacid (not indicated, but known).

SUMMARY The total genetic complement of a human gamete corresponds to over 3,000 million nucleotides (3,000 Megabases), partitioned into 22 chromosomes of different size, 1 sex chromosome (X or Y) and many copies of small-sized (16.6 Kilobases) mitochondrial DNA. Each zygote, resulting from fertilization, is endowed with a double complement, one conveyed by the sperm and one contributed by the female gamete. Cytoplasm, including the whole set of mitochondria, is almost completely contributed by the maternal gamete. Thus, a novel individual has two copies for each chromosome, one fron the father and the other from the mother, while mitochondrial DNA is exclusively maternal. Only about 3% of human DNA corresponds to coding sequences, i.e. to segments which can be transcribed into RNAs used as such (i.e. ribosomal RNAs and transfer RNAs), or transcribed to messenger RNAs and then translated into proteins. According to current estimates, the number of human genes (i.e. DNA sequences encoding products) is probably less than 40,000.   ->

A typical gene includes a regulatory sequence and a number of coding sequences, called "exons", interrupted by long non-coding sequences, called "introns". Gene size and number of exons is very variable from gene to gene. Few genes are intronless.

At each cell division, DNA is replicated. During replication, random errors occur. Additional errors may derive from physical and chemical mutagenesis. Such errors are the origin of DNA variations in somatic and in germ cells. Consequent variations (mutations) in coding sequences may alter the aminoacid sequence of the corresponding products and may result in functional defects at cellular level. Deletion or duplication of large stretches of DNA may also occur and may lead to alteration of gene dosage. About 4% of human gametes presumably carry at least one novel mutation in one of the genes, in each generation.

About of 97% of human genomic DNA has no coding function and it is particularly rich in repetitive sequences of different length. Mutations in such sequences produce variations in the number of repeats. Such DNA variants can be used as "DNA markers" when attempting to trace the transmission of a given DNA segment from generation to generation.

Individual genomes show high variability in coding and in non-coding sequences. At each meiosis, additional variability results from recombination between segments of homologous chromosomes, giving rise to novel haplotypes.

CHAPTER 2

FROM GENOME TO CLINICAL PHENOTYPE

2.1 Analyzing the human transcriptome

In general, human genes are differentially expressed in space (different tissues) and time (different age during lifespan, but also different time in every single day), possibly with the exception of those (the so-called "housekeeping genes") coding for products involved in general functions of all cell types. Many genes produce tissue-specific or stage-specific isoforms, by tissue-specific promoters or by tissue-specific alternative splicing.

The whole set of transcripts released by the genome in a cell or in a tissue at a given time is called "transcriptome".

In the last ten years, three different methods (ESTs sequencing, SAGE and cDNA microarrays) enabled researchers to investigate human transcriptome.

The first step of this revolutionary approach was the possibility of extracting RNA from a selected tissue and of obtaining from it a cDNA (complementary DNA), by reverse transcription (i.e. DNA synthesis from an RNA template, catalyzed by reverse transcriptase).

The second step was to understand that short sequences of cDNA, obtained by its random fragmentation, are actually "tags" of genes which produced the mRNAs from which cDNAs were retro-transcribed. Therefore, by sequencing random samples of a mixture of fragments of cDNAs obtained from a given tissue, it would be possible to identify which genes are active in such a tissue, provided the DNA sequence of every human gene would be known. On the other hand, finding a segment of cDNA sequence with no match with any known human gene would immediately denounce the presence of a still unknown human gene transcript.

This reasoning prompted C. Venter in 1991 to start sequencing ESTs (Expressed Sequence Tags) (Figure 2.1) and to establish a database of ESTs. (Adams, 1992; 1993).

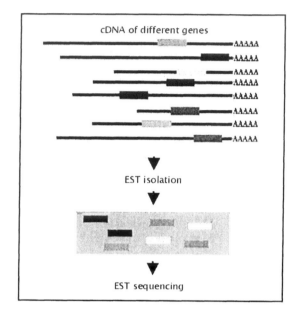

Figure 2.1: ESTs sequencing. The sequencing of random segments of cDNA molecules (obtained by retro-transcription of a mixture of mRNAs extracted from a tissue) would identify single trancripts and would produce a reliable representation of the composition of the original cDNA library (from SAGE website, modified)

Venter's method underwent a further improvement in 1992, by K. Okubo, who selected to "cut" the tail of each cDNA by aid of the restriction enzyme MboI and to sequence only this 3' end segment, about 250 nt long, which they called "gene signature". In this way every sequenced segment of cDNA corresponded to a single transcript, while in Venter's procedure a single transcript could produce multiple ESTs. The differences between the two methods are illustrated in Fig. 2.2.

After Venter's and OKubo's enterprises, many laboratories started projects of ESTs sequencing of different human tissues, with the goal of detecting (and eventually patenting) unknown human genes relevant to medicine.

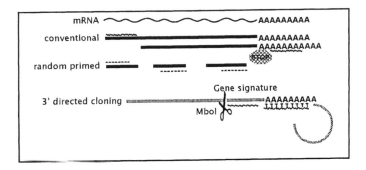

Figure 2.2: Different methods for obtaining ESTs from cDNA molecules. Conventional (after C.Venter) method involves random fragmentation of cDNA molecules; alternatively, ESTs may be obtained by randomly primed cDNA synthesis, while K. Okubo's method isolates only 3'-end ESTs, called "gene signatures" (from BODYMAP website).

Most of the huge amount of data generated by these projects was subsequently collected in a public database (dbEST) at NCBI (National Center for Biological Information); however, some data concerning tissues of potential interest for biotechnology industry, owned by private databases, remained inaccessible.

Later, a novel database was developed, called UniGene (http://www.ncbi.nlm.nih.gov/UniGene/), a catalogue of all ESTs available on public domain. In this database all available ESTs are compared to each other and grouped into "UniGene Clusters". Each UniGene cluster in the catalogue, corresponding to a putative transcript of a human gene, is fully annotated and directly linked to other relevant genomic databases. Until February 2001, when the first draft of the complete DNA sequence of human genome was made accessible on-line (Lander, 2001;Venter, 2001), UniGene represented the most versatile and useful tool for identification of human genes. With its

34

over 96,000 cluster sets, including over 3,011,282 ESTs sequences, UniGene, maintained at NCBI, is still the main human gene indexing database.

In 1995, V.E. Velculescu devised a novel method, called SAGE (Sequential Analysis of Gene Expression), with the aim of analyzing transcriptional profiles of single human tissues and accelerating the discovery of novel genes. The method, shown in Figure 2.3, is derived by EST sequencing, but it has the advantage of considerably reducing time and cost of the sequencing effort.

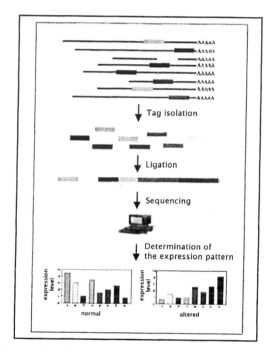

Figure 2.3 : SAGE (Sequential Analysis of Gene Expression)
(from SAGE website)

The principle on which SAGE is based is that a very high number ($4^9 =$ 262,144) of different oligonucleotides 9-nt long may be obtained. Therefore, there is a good probability that one given 9-nt oligonucleotide might unambiguously match a single transcript sequence. Like ESTs, such a short oligonucleotides might be considered "tags" of the corresponding transcript sequences. In practice, cDNAs obtained from a given tissue are cut into "tags" by a specific restriction enzyme (usually NIaIII). After undergoing a second cut by a different restriction enzyme and several manipulations, tags are linked together in long concatamers.

Each tag is separated from the preceding and from the following tags by short spacers of 4 nucleotides. DNA sequencing of concatamers will identify the sequence of all tags and computer analysis will reveal the correspondence between tags and transcripts. Automation of this process ensures a quick identification of all tags, their annotation and computation of the relative frequency of each tag. Tags not corresponding to known transcripts would be immediately detected.

Although tag-to-gene correspondence is not always as precise as expected, SAGE is an efficient method for obtaining the transcriptional profile of a tissue. A database of SAGE results is available as a section of UniGene.

More recently, a novel method, based on hybridization of cDNA molecules on DNA microarrays (Fig. 2.4) gained popularity among researchers. The principle of this technique (Schena, 1995) is simple: a series of double-stranded cDNA are immobilized in a given order (array) on a solid surface. By use of a robotic station, aliquots of DNA samples (each corresponding to a given gene) are spotted on a glass or plastic surface. The position of each DNA sample is automatically recorded. After having been labeled with a fluorescent marker, a mixture of cDNA molecules obtained by retrotranscription from the selected tissue is hybridized to the array. Mini-spots of fluorescence are detected in correspondence of single points of the array, by laser scanning. Results are automatically transformed into digital outputs and analyzed by statistical software.

In reality each array is hybridized both with test cDNA and with control cDNA, marked with different fluorescent markers. Competitive hybridization reveals which transcripts are more abundant or more rare than expected in the test tissue, i.e, which genes are differentially expressed in the selected experimental condition.

36

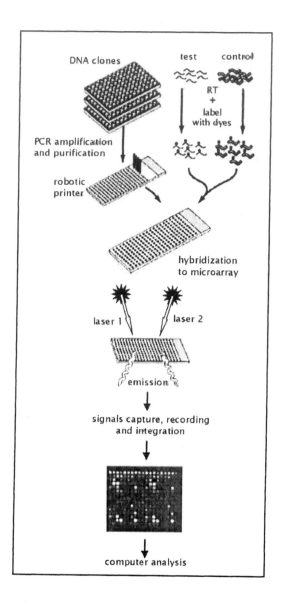

Fig.2.4: An experiment using a cDNA array
(by courtesy of Dr. G. Lanfranchi)

Although cDNA arrays technology is very reliable, the exceedingly large mass of data obtained in each single experiment (resulting from thousands of genes) often make statistical analysis problematic.

Moreover, large inter- and intra-experiment variation in hybridization signals, due to unknown variables or to poorly controlled conditions, poses additional problems.

Several softwares are available for efficiently performing such analyses, based on different statistics, but, as a rule-of-thumb, genes showing more than two-fold expression in the experimental condition than in the control (or vice versa), may be reasonably assumed as differentially expressed.

DNA microchips technology was originally developed to detect and identify short sequences of DNA, on the basis of their hybridization to short oligonucleotide sequences linked to a solid substrate (in origin a silicon chip, from which the name "DNA chip").

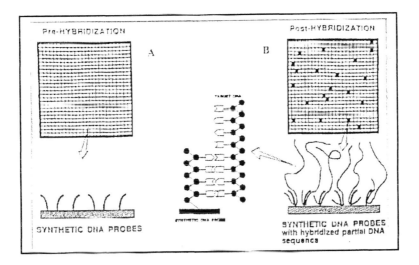

Fig. 2.5: Principles of the DNA-chip technology. A) In-situ DNA synthesis takes place, due to photoactivation of selected points, in presence of a solution containing a given nucleotide (e.g. T). After washing out, solution is changed (e.g. with G). Synthesis will occur only in points subjected to activation, following programmed masking and unmasking of different points. B) Hybridization of target DNA to synthetic DNA probes.

Photolithographic masks are designed by computer algorythms, in order to define the exposure of each single point of the "chip" surface. Then, oligonucleotides (called "probes") are chemically synthetized on each single spot, by aid of photochemical reactions occurring on the unmasked points (Fig. 2.5). By this technology, high-density arrays of probes may generated, each specific oligo having a pre-defined position in the array. The nucleic acid to be analyzed (called "target molecule") is amplified and labeled by a fluorescent reporter molecule. Labeled targets are then hybridized to the array of probes and sites of hybridization detected by a laser scanner. Since position of each probe on the array is known, the identity of the molecule which hybridized to it can be determined by complementarity.

The great advantage of DNA microchips is the possibility of arraying half a million oligonucleotide probes, corresponding to aproximately 12,000 genes, on about 1 square inch. In the next future DNA microchips and DNA microarrays will be used not only for research, but also for diagnosis (Pastinene, 1997). Actually, at the very end, any disease may be cosidered, at cellular and tissue level, an alteration of the normal transcriptional profile. Therefore, once specific alterations of the transcriptional profile of a given tissue could be unequivocably ascribed to a given disease, such alterations, revealed by DNA chips or cDNA arrays, could become diagnostic. Equally, DNA microarrays could enable to monitor the eventual remediation of such alterations, produced by treatment. Endomyocardial biopsy proved to be a suitable, safe and ethically acceptable method for monitoring biological condition of transplanted hearts. Therefore, we might envisage the use of endomyocardial biopsies for DNA microarray analyses.

2.2 The differential expression of human genes

All human cells have the same set of genes. Thus, structural and functional differences among cells and tissues must be ascribed to differential transcription (expression) of selected genes.

It is widely accepted that in each cell only a relatively small fraction of human genes are expressed at a given time. Most of them are expressed at very low level, contributing to whole transcription only with few copies of mRNA. Probably less than 10,000 genes (i.e. 25% of the total) are expressed at detectable level in a given differentiated human tissue at a given time. Differential transcription of genes implies the existence of controls.

Control of gene expression may operate in each step of the transfer of genetic information from DNA to proteins, but in higher organisms it is mainly exerted at the level of transcription, i.e. synthesis of mRNAs.

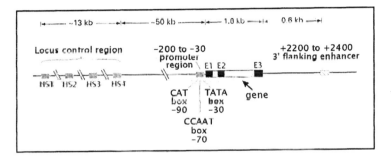

Figure 2.6: Schematic representation of a gene with its major control regions (from Strachan, modified)

Control of transcription is mostly performed by specific molecules ("transcription factors"), able to bind DNA in correspondence of specific sequences ("regulatory sequences"). Regulatory DNA sequences are mostly in the region upstream the initiation of trancription of each gene (Fig. 2.6).

They include the so-called "core promoter" (from-45 to +40 from the transcription initiation site), the "promoter region" (from -50 to –200, including positive and negative regulators, enhancers and silencers) and "response elements". Moreover, other regulative DNA sequences (LCR = Locus Control Region) can be found several Kbs upstream the initiation site.

Several transcription factors are tissue-specific. Binding of transcription factors to double stranded DNA molecule modifies its curvature, in proximity of the initiation point, thus enabling the complex of RNA polymerase to "land" on the DNA and to start its process.

A schematic view of complex interactions involved in transcription is given in Fig. 2.7.

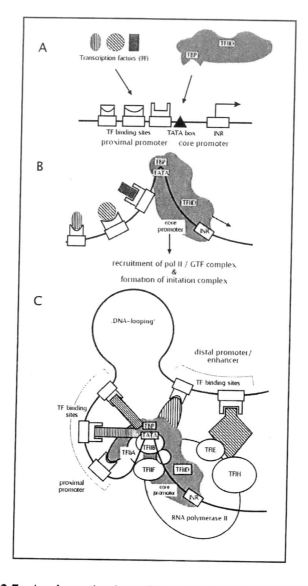

Fig. 2.7: A schematic view of the initiation of transcription.
(From Werner, modified)

Transcription factors are product of other genes, which, in turn, may be under control of other transcription factors produced by other genes. Therefore, the expression of some genes may generate a cascade of activation affects.

In general, genes expressed at the same time in the same cell (co-expressed) are often co-regulated, i.e. under the same control.

Transcription in specific genes may be induced by hormones, growth factors and by cellular messengers (e.g. cyclic AMP) acting on response elements.

Transcriptional activity of genome in a given cell or tissue at a given time should be viewed as a part of a very complex network of interactions between the genome and its environment, resulting, in turn, from the interactions between intracellular and extracellular environment.

A "genomic response" would take place in response to any biochemical perturbation which, directly or indirectly, could be able to act on transcription of one or more genes.

2.3 From transcriptome to proteome and metabolome

After having being transcribed from selected segments of DNA, messenger RNAs undergo maturation and then they are translated into proteins by ribosomes. Newly synthetized proteins may undergo post-translational modifications, such as cleavage, glycosylation, phosphorylation, and so on.

Due to extensive usage of alternative promoters and alternative splicing, probably over 250,000 different proteins are potentially coded by our genes However their number could be possibly much larger, if we consider potential proteins deriving from post-translational modifications.

The entire set of proteins of a particular cell or tissue is called "proteome". Two-dimensional electrophoretic separation (Fig.2.8), followed by elution of single protein spots and by their analysis by mass spectrometry is able to identify each single protein of the original mixture, thus providing

42

information on the real final product of the release of genetic information from the genome. This research approach is particularly important, after the description of human coding DNA sequences is almost completed. We just entered the "post-genomic" era, i.e. the era of investigations on transcriptomes and proteomes.

All proteins produced by genome expression are "contained" in the cell. In reality they are constituent of the cell, where, through their interactions, they form structures, compartments and chains of biochemical reactions. Part of cellular proteins are secreted and released in the extracellular environment, where they may act as signals.

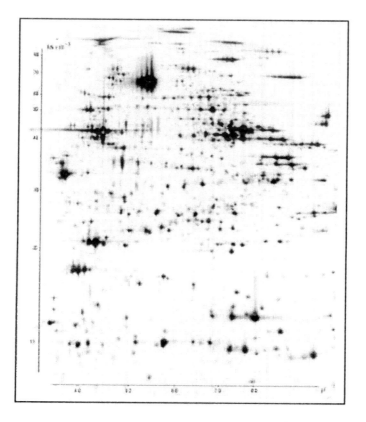

Figure 2.8: Two-dimensional separation of proteins from human heart, by sodium-duodecyl-sulphate polyacrylamide gel electrophoresis.

The set of proteins participating in a complex metabolic network is called "metabolome".

Presently, the model of organization of metabolic networks is a so-called "scale-free" network model (Fig. 2.9). Individual proteins are considered as elements in a network of protein-protein interactions, with a specific function within functional modules. Connectivity between elements (nodes) of the network would be mainly maintained by a few highly connected nodes, whose removal would drastically alter the network topology, whereas errors or attacks involving the majority of nodes with small connectivity should not alter the path structure of the remaining nodes, thus having no impact on the overall network structure.

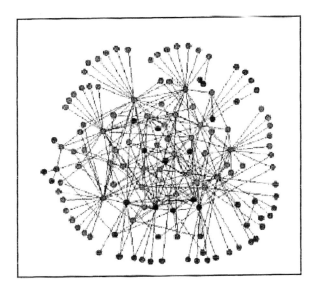

Fig. 2.9: Representation of "scale-free" model of a metabolic network (see text for details) (From Alberts, modified)

Recent data, derived from investigations by cDNA microarrays and DNA-chips, suggest that differentiated state of human tissues is characterized by high expression of a limited number of genes and by low or very low

44

transcription of many genes. Multiple-tag experiments revealed the key role of relatively small groups of genes with similar expression, probably functionally related and possibly co-regulated. Highly expressed genes are expected to produce high concentrations of the corresponding proteins. For stoichiometric reasons, such proteins would have high probability of interacting with several other proteins, thus becoming relevant nodes of the metabolic network. Therefore, upregulation of a limited number of genes could force a given differentiated cell to maintain its stable structural and functional phenotype during time, i.e, unless it would be subjected to strong perturbations affecting transcription levels of genes coding for functional nodes of such network.

2.4 The transcriptome of the human heart

The first compendium of genes expressed in the cardiovascular system was produced by Hwang in 1997 (Tab. 2.1).

Table 2.1: An estimate of relative distribution of functions among genes active in the human cardiovascular systems (according to Hwang, 1997)

Functional category	No. of genes	%
Cell division	260	5.68
Cell signalling	836	18.27
Cell structure and motility	443	9.68
Cell defense	307	6.71
Gene expression	1,907	23.97
Metabolism	717	15.67
Unclassified	915	20.00

More recently, a small subset of such catalogue appeared in a publication by the same Author, where the correspondence of in silico predictions with experimental data on gene expression in heart was demonstrated (Hwang, 2000).

Data on genomic expression in adult human cardiac tissue may be retrieved from the Okubo's "BodyMap" website, where the expression of genes in atria and ventricles are reported separately. Most data reported in this database derive from the original work of Okubo's group (http://bodymap.ims.u-tokyo.ac.jp).

CaGE (The Cardiac Gene Expression Knowledgebase) maintained at the John Hopkins University (http://cyrus.wbmei.jhu.edu/) is a gene-centric knowledgebase designed to serve as web-based reference for physicians and scientists interested in gene expression in human cardiac tissue. It includes data found in the web and experimental data on expression profiles of human heart failure.

A catalogue of genes expressed in heart was also obtained by applying a bioinformatic and computational approach to UniGene data (Bortoluzzi, 2000). This catalogue which is available on public domain (http://telethon.bio.unipd.it/bioinfo/HGXP/), includes over 2,000 genes with their estimated level of expression.

It is important to notice that original data derived from ESTs sequencing, as well as data derived from bioinformatic reconstruction of transcriptional profile of the adult human heart, suffer from an important bias: they refer not to myocardiocytes, but to cardiac tissue, which include coronary vessels and different cell types. On the other hand, in order to get a reasonably good representation of transcripts in the sample of cDNA obtained from myocardium, the specimen should correspond to not less than 50 milligrams of fresh tissue. This implies unavoidable contamination by endothelial cells, lymphocytes, fibroblasts and so on. Laser-capture microdissection is a more sophisticated and precise method, but the limited size of the sample greatly reduces the probability of detecting cDNA corresponding to weakly expressed genes, even if SAGE would be applied.

Future development of diagnostic approaches based on cDNA microarrays and DNA-chips technologies would suffer by the same limitation, since also in these cases one must rely on biopsies, i.e. tissue samples of small or very small size .

At present, it is possible to monitor with high confidence only variations in the expression of a limited number of genes which appear highly expressed in the heart (Barrans, 2001). The distinction between genes expressed in myocardial cells and those active in coronary vessels or in other cells of cardiac tissue is at the moment impossible; however data on differential gene expression in different components of the heart may be obtained from alternative sources (in-situ RT-PCR, immunohistochemical staining, etc).

According to the scale-free network model of the cellular transcriptome and metabolome (see section 2.3, this chapter), relevant phenotypical alterations at tissue level should depend on significant modification of the expression in a relatively small number of genes; present methods seem to be able to detect them.

In conclusion, analyzing transcriptional profile of cardiac tissue promises to be very interesting and helpful.

2.5 Genotype and phenotype

At the beginning of the development of Genetics, researchers adopted the term "phenotype" to refer to observable characteristics of an individual organism, or cell. Phenotype was considered to be determined by "genotype", i.e. the genetic constitution of the individual organism or cell. Later, experimental evidences forced the researchers to modify their definition of phenotype by saying that an individual organism or cell results from the interaction of its genotype with the environment (Fig 2.10).

Actually, there are conditions, called "phenocopies", due to environmental factors acting on genotype and producing an appearance similar to that corresponding to a different genotype. For instance, forty years ago, the administration of thalidomide to pregnant women induced in fetuses phocomely (severe malformations of limbs), a rare condition reported as genetically determined.

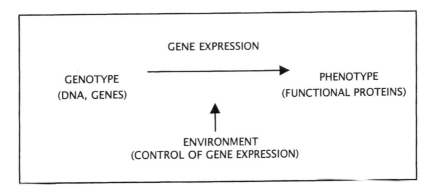

Figure 2.10: Relationships between genotype, phenotype and environment. Environmental factors may exert a direct or indirect control on gene expression.

For one century, human genetics strove to identify genetic determinants of human disease, by identifying and describing "abnormal" phenotypes and by reconstructing patterns of their inheritance in families.

This approach was very successful in the second half of last century, leading to identification and description of several hundreds of diseases inherited as "simple traits" (the so-called "mendelian disorders") and to their genetic mapping (localization of the involved gene on a specific chromosomal segment), much earlier than DNA sequence of the human genome was produced. For such diseases, the relationships between genotype (i.e. mutational variation in a single "gene") and phenotype (clinical features) are relatively simple.

Mutation in a gene could produce a reduced amount of mRNA or a mRNA carrying a modification in its sequence. Translation of such an altered mRNA would produce a protein modified in its sequence and function. Functional alteration of a single protein or, alternatively, a reduction in its amount due to genetically defective gene expression might be harmful to the functional module to which the protein participate in the metabolic network of the cell or the the series of interactions between proteins producing the cytoskeleton and the chains of signals transduction.

A classical example is given by the well-known relationship between mutation in the gene coding for phenylalanine hydroxylase and Phenylketonuria (PKU). This disease is inherited as autosomal recessive trait. When a zygote receive one mutant (defective) gene copy from each of the parents, a fetus will develop, carrying the mutation (defect) in homozygosis. The baby will show an inborn defect of metabolism, because of a single defective biochemical reaction. Actually, his defective phenylalanine hydroxylase is unable to convert phenylalanine into tyrosine. Cells can obtain tyrosine from an alternative metabolic source, and phenylalanine can be metabolized to phenyl-pyruvic acid. However, this reaction is not efficient enough to avoid an abnormal and progressive accumulation of phenyl-pyruvic acid, which degradation product, phenylketone, is excreted in the urine (phenylketonuria, from which the name given to the disease). High concentrations of phenyl-pyruvic acid are toxic for neurons, producing a severe brain damage. Fortunately, early dietary treatment (strong reduction of phenylalanine supply) after having detected the condition in the newborn, proved effective in reducing the pathogenic consequences of the mutation. This example says that knowing molecular pathogenesis would, in theory, enable to devise a corrective treatment for any genetic disease (Fig. 2.11).

Unfortunately, in most cases our knowledge is too limited to help in this matter. However, the situation is likely to change favourably in the next future, due to increasing progress in understanding human biochemistry and molecular cell biology.

Coming back to genetic diseases, we know that some mutations are inherited as dominant traits, while other as recessive. The distinction is made by analyzing the phenotype of the heterozygote, i.e. the subject who carries in every cell one normal copy (normal allele) and one mutant copy (mutant allele) of the gene involved in the observed phenotype.

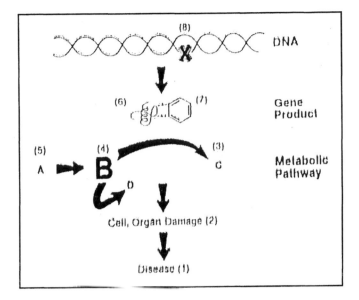

Fig. 2.11: Cascade of effects from gene mutation to phenotype level. A pathogenic DNA mutation (8) reflects in a protein alteration, which affects its functional properties. In most cases altered protein function is the cause of perturbation of one or more metabolic pathways. Being genetic in nature, the defect will be present in all cells of the same tissue. Therefore, a tissue damage (2) is expected. If this damage is relevant enough, it could reflect in the functional alteration of an organ, a system and of the whole organism (1). Present therapeutic strategies mostly involve administration of drugs (for correcting the defect at biochemical level (6,7) dietary restrictions (4,5) or supplementations (3). In the most severe cases, organ transplantation may be the only choice, like in cardiomyopathies at advanced stage. Future therapeutic strategies could involve the administration of drugs to activate or inhibit the transcription of selected genes, or the administration of copies of normal genes, in order to restore normal function.

Let us assume that the subject carrying two mutant alleles (homozygote mutant) shows a peculiar disease and that the subject carrying two normal (also called "wild-type") alleles (homozygote normal) doesn't show any sign of such disease. Now, let's consider a subject who carries one normal and one mutant allele (heterozygote). If this subject shows signs of the disease like the homozygote for the mutant allele, we might deduce that the disease is

50

inherited as "dominant" trait, while, if the heterozygote would be healthy, the trait should be inherited as "recessive".

In reality, the decision if a given disease is inherited as a dominant or as a recessive trait is taken after studies on many families, by a statistical approach called "Segregation analysis" and developed by N.E. Morton in 1959.

In clinical practice it is not infrequent to observe that in a family with recurrence of a dominant disease some subjects having one parent and one sib affected (thus being obligate carriers of the mutant allele), do not show signs of the disease. In this cases the trait is said having a "incomplete" or "reduced" penetrance in family. An example of such situation is shown in Fig. 2.12.

Reduced penetrance is mostly attributable to the effects of differences in individual genetic background. In cardiac disorders, often an age-related penetrance is observed, probably related to progressive accumulation of myocardial damages with time.

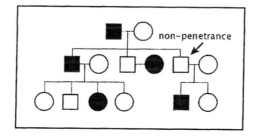

Figure 2.12 : A family tree in which a dominant disease trait shows reduced penetrance (on the right side, an obligate carrier of the mutant allele appears unaffected).

2.6 Molecular explanation of dominance of some mutations

Some gene mutations are inherited as dominant traits, other as recessives. Dominance and recessivity have their explanation at molecular level , as shown in Fig. 2.13.

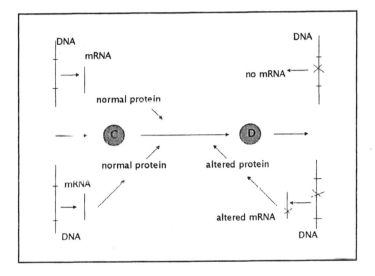

Figure 2.13: Explanation of dominance and recessivity at molecular level. Two possible situations are depicted: a) mutation suppressing mRNA synthesis (e.g. regulatory mutation, gene deletion, etc); b) mutation modifying the protein sequence (e.g. a missense mutation). The gene coding for a protein involved in a metabolic step (from M to N) is in heterozygosis (normal/mutant)

Every somatic cell is diploid, i.e. it carries two copies (homologues) for each chromosome. Therefore, a cell will have two copies of the same gene (alleles), except for genes carried by sex chromosomes.

A normal allele would produce, at its correct level of expression, a normal mRNA, which, in turn, will be regularly processed and translated into protein. This protein would then undergo correct post-translational modifications, thus becoming fully functional.

Many different mutations are possible (see table 1.2, Chapter 1), but, in practical terms, only two situations to be considered: a) mutant allele gives origin to no protein; b) mutant allele produces a modified protein.

Case a will produce a "dosage effect". In fact, in the heterozygote intracellular concentration of the protein coded by the considered gene will be reduced by one half. If cells could be able to maintain a normal function, in spite of the reduced levels of such a protein, such a mutation would behave as a recessive, since no alteration in the phenotype would be observed at cellular, tissue or clinical level.

On the other hand, if cells would need for their normal functioning a relatively high level of such protein, reduced dosage, due to mutation, would be harmful and adverse effects would be observed in the heterozygote, thus evidencing the dominant effect of the mutation. This reasoning applies also to mutations in regulatory sequences, which may reduce or abolish transcription of a given gene.

In case b, mutation may produce a truncated protein (nonsense and frame-shift mutations). If truncated protein is quickly degraded, the resulting situation is very similar to that of case a.

On the other hand, if a mutation produces a change in the aminoacid sequence, the resulting protein may show different functional properties. If mutation implies a loss-of-function, dominance or recessivity of the mutation will depend on the cellular need of the protein product. It is interesting to notice that cells of different tissues may have different needs, therefore a mutation may manifest its effects in one tissue, but not in others.

Because of a missense mutation, a protein may acquire a novel functional property (gain-of-function). If the "novel" protein would induce in the metabolic network a considerable alteration, a dominant effect is expected. In fact, many dominant mutations correspond to situations of "gain-of-function".

Since the effects of a dominant mutation overcomes those of the normal allele, often the terms "dominant negative" or "toxic gain-of-function" (with reference to the harmful effect on cell metabolism) are used. Moreover, the normal allele is considered "haploinsufficient" since a single copy of it is insufficient to produce a normal phenotype.

In many cases, proteins are active in cells as multimers, i.e. complexes made by a certain number of identical (homomultimers) or diferent (heteromultimers) molecules. In the heterozygote, mutant copies of a protein would be equally included in multimers, as normal copies do. For instance, cardiac ryanodine receptor is a complex made of four copies of RyR2 protein, associated with four FKBP12.6 units, to form the functional ryanodine receptor. In heterozygotes for a RyR2 missense mutations, some receptors will be made by four normal RyR2 molecules, some by four mutant RyR2 proteins, while the majority would be made by mixtures of normal and mutant proteins.

Some mutations may increase the activity of enzymes or their affinity for the normal substrate. Also in these cases, a disturbance in a biochemical pathway is expected.

Mutations in regulatory sequences may cause expression of given genes in wrong cells or tissues, or in the wrong time (gain-of-function). In some cases, different mutations in the same gene may correspond to different diseases: mutations. Different mutations of the same gene not only may produce different diseases, but they may even produce diseases showing different modes of inheritance. For instance, some mutations of the gene KVLQT1 cause Long -QT syndrome and are inherited as dominant trait, while other mutations of the same gene are inherited as recessive traits and, in homozygosis, they cause Jervell and Lange-Nielsen syndrome.

2.7 Gene dosage

In human somatic cells, every chromosome is present in two copies (the so-called "homologues").

Sex cromosomes are homologous in females (XX) but heterologous in males (XY). Chromosome X and chromosome Y are different in size and in gene content, although they share homologous DNA sequences. The apparent disequilibrium between gene dosage in males and females is compensated for by hypercondensation of large part of one copy of the X chromosome, which prevents the transcription of genes included in such regions. For many genes located on chromosome X, only one copy is active in female somatic cells. Inactivation is a random and irreversible process, therefore one X chromosome will be "inactive" in some cells but not in others. Heterozygotes for gene(s) located in a chromosomal region subjected to inactivation, may show alternative cellular phenotypes (normal or mutant) within the same tissue. This phenomenon is a kind of "somatic mosaicism".

In males there is not a real homologous counterpart of X chromosome. Therefore, mutations in genes carried by X chromosome (X-linked) will be always expressed in males, regardless they are dominant or recessive. Since males have only one copy of the X chromosome, these mutations are said to be expressed in "hemizygosis" (which means: half of the dose typical of the zygote)

The phenomenon of X-chromosome inactivation points at the importance of the correct dosage for every gene. This is confirmed by the fact that in the human genome some genes are active as a single copy. The other copy (in some genes the paternal, in others the maternal copy) is inactivated by "genomic imprinting" and not accessible to transcription. In each generation, "old" imprinting is erased in germline cells and the new, sex-specific imprinting is established, in female germline during oocyte maturation and in male in the primary spermatocyte.

Correct gene dosage of an individual may be altered because of deletions or duplications of chromosomal regions. A gross disequilibrium in gene dosage occurs when entire chromosomes are duplicated (like in trisomics) or lost (like in monosomics). In these cases (e.g. Turner syndrome, Down syndrome etc.) clinical phenotype shows multi-systemic affection, due to alteration of gene dosage in many genes and consequent pathogenic effect in many tissues.

Alterations of gene dosage may occur in somatic cells of some tissues, because of polyploidy, i.e. multiplication of the normal DNA complement, due to replication not followed by cell division.

In most mammalian species cardiomyocytes have two nuclei, i.e. a dosage of genes double than normal. In humans, over 90% of cardiac myocytes are mononucleated, but with age some of them may become polyploid and may show as much as 8-fold the normal DNA content.

2.8 Peculiarity of phenotypes due to mutations in mitochondrial DNA

Pathogenic mutations in genes carried by mytochondrial DNA are well documented. They mostly affect SNC and skeletal muscle, but cardiological affections (hypetrophic cardiomyopathy, dilated cardiomyopathy, heart block, pre-excitation syndrome) are also reported in the literature.

Each human somatic cell harbours more than 1000 molecules of mtDNA, derived from those of the mytochondria of the zygote.

Mitochondria undergo division by fission, independently of the timing of cell division; replicates of mtDNA are distributed among the newly formed mitochondria and, at each cell division, mitochondria are distributed between the two daughter cells, at random.

Mutations occur in mtDNA more frequently than in nuclear DNA, since mtDNA is exposed to a rather mutagenic environment (peroxides are very abundant within the mitochondrion) and it lacks associated nucleoproteins and efficient repair systems.

A mutation in mtDNA will be propagated through the genealogy of mitochondria, thus each cell could contain a mixture or mutant and non-mutant mitochondria. Because of random sorting of mitochondria in daughter cells, in theory one cell might receive mitochondria containing an almost pure population of mutant or normal mtDNA molecule. This situation would be referred as "homoplasmy", while "heteroplasmy" corresponds to a heterogeneous population of mutant and non-mutant mtDNA molecules.

The number of mtDNA molecules undergo reduction ("mitochondrial genetic bottleneck"), before being amplified to the very large amount in the mature oocyte. Because reduction is a random process, the proportion of mutant vs non-mutant mtDNA molecules may greatly vary among oocytes. Then, all children from a woman heteroplasmic for a mtDNA mutation would inherit mutant mtDNA molecules, but the proportion of such mutant DNA molecules could be very different from individual to individual. Moreover, since phenotypic expression of a mtDNA mutation depends on relative proportion of normal and mutant mtDNA (threshold effect) in cells of different tissues, pleiotropy and large variability in clinical phenotypes corresponding to mtDNA mutations is almost the rule.

In Kearns-Sayre syndrome (KSS), a large deletion in the mtDNA causes progressive external ophtalmoplegia with heart-block. In other mitochondrial diseases, some subjects may show a severe encephalopathy, while others, in the same sibship, may manifest diabetes and deafness. Intrafamiliar variability is paralleled by inter-familiar variance.

The most common mtDNA mutation (A3243G, in gene coding for tRNA for leucine) in usually associated with MELAS (Myoclonic Epilepsy,Lactic Acidosis, Stroke), but in some families it may predominantly cause diabetes and deafness, while in others it produces cardiomyopathy.

2.9 Multi-factorial diseases

Several congenital malformations and many common disorders of the adults age cannot be ascribed to a defect in a single gene. However, familiar concentration of cases points to a genetic component. It is widely accepted that such diseases may result from a combination of mutations in different genes, none of which determining a specific disease, and from environmental factors, which could trigger the development of the disease, accelerate its progression or increase its severity.

In industrialized countries, the impact of multifactorial diseases on human population is estimated to be about 60%.

The genetic ground of multifactorial diseases is polygenic inheritance. Let's assume that two independent genes (A and B), are potentially involved in a cardiac affection, since both code for proteins relevant to cardiac function. For simplicity, we postulate for each of them a normal allele (respectively A and B) and a mutant allele (respectively A' and B') producing a small dysfunction, but not a disease.

As shown in Tab. 2.2, the cross between two heterozygotes (AA',BB' x AA',BB') would produce 16 different possible genotypes in their progeny, as a result of the independent assortment of the different alleles.

Table 2.2: Possible genotypes resulting in the progeny of a parent heterozygous in two genes, carried by two different chromosomes, e.g. gene A by chromosome 4 and gene B by chromosome 15 (see text for explanation)

gametes	A, B	A', B	A, B	A', B'
A, B	A A, B B	A A', B B	A A, B B'	A A', B B'
A', B	A'A, B B	A'A', B B	A'A, B B'	A'A', B B'
A, B'	A A, B B'	A A', B'B	A A, B'B'	A A', B'B'
A', B'	A'A, B'B	A'A', B'B	A'A, B'B'	A'A', B'B'
gametes	A, B	A', B	A, B'	A', B'
A, B	A A, B B	A A', B B	A A, B B'	A A', B B'

There will be only 1/16 chance that an individual in the progeny could be free of any mutant allele (AA,BB) or could carry both mutant alleles (A'A',B'B').

In the cross of the heterozygote with a homozygote for normal alleles (AA',BB' x AA,BB) the heterozygote would produce four different types of gametes (A,B; A',B; A,B', a'B'), while the homozygote would produce only a single type of gametes (A,B). None of the possible siblings could become homozygote for both mutant alleles.

Let's suppose that genotype A'A',B'B' (homozygote for mutant allels in both genes) is at high risk of developing a cardiac affection in the normal environment, while AA,BB (homozygote for normal alleles in both genes) have no chance of developing such cardiac affection, unless exposed to peculiar and rare environmental factors. The other possible genotypes (AA',BB; AA,BB'; AA',BB'; A'A',BB'; AA',B'B') will have different levels of risk to develop the affection in absence of peculiar environmental factors, according to their individual dosage of mutant alleles. In fact, some subjects carrying mutations in the considered genes might develop the affection, but it will be difficult to establish a clear causal relationship with their genetic status, because of the confounding effect of individual biological histories, i.e. the differential exposure to environmental risk factors.

Therefore, we should conclude that mutations in these genes may pre-dispose to the development of such affection, although a precise risk assessment would be very difficult.

Fig. 2.14 shows the combined effects of genetic and environmental factors on the distribution of risk of developing the disease in the general population. In the figure, a sharp threshold is marked, over which the disease is supposed to develop. In realty, thresholds are never so sharp. Moreover, in most models the effects of single mutations and of single environmental factors are taken as additive, while in reality often they are multiplicative, or additive in some instances and multiplicative in others.

Most genetic models of multifactorial diseases consider a very limited number of genes. This oversimplification may appear inappropriate, in front of the very large number of genes possibly involved. However, the development of a multifactorial disease is believed to be due to the effect of mutation on a limited number of genes, with rather relevant effect ("major genes").

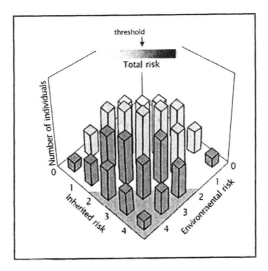

Figure 2.14: Combined effects of genetic and environmental contribution to the development of a multifactorial disease. On the x axis the environmental risk is plotted, on the z axis the relative number of subjects falling in the same category of genetic and environmental risk. Severity of risk is indicated by dark gray.

Manifestation of cardiovascular diseases is influenced by other phenotypes related to quantitative traits, as blood pressure, body weight, and so on. Identifying loci corresponding to major genes involved in such traits (QTL, Quantitative Trait Loci) is one great challenge of the present genomic research.

SUMMARY All human cells have the same set of genes. However, in each cell only a relatively small fraction of genes, probably less than 25% of the total, are expressed at detectable level at a given time. Structural and functional differences among cells are due to differential expression of selected genes, controlled through interaction of specific proteins with regulative DNA sequences, mostly located in a region, encompassing less than 1,000 nucleotides, upstream the initiation of transcription of each gene. Genes expressed at the same time in the same cell are often co-regulated, i.e. under the same control.

For in-vitro analysis of genome expression, cellular messenger-RNAs may be artificially transcribed to complementary DNA (cDNA). cDNA is hybridized to arrays of DNA molecules corresponding to segments of specific coding sequences. In this way, qualitative and quantitative analysis of genomic transcription in a given tissue is possible. Data showed that a genomic response, in terms of gene expression, takes place in response to many biochemical perturbations and, in particular, to hormones and intracellular messengers acting on response elements at DNA level. After having being transcribed from selected genes, messenger RNAs undergo maturation and they are then translated into proteins. Due to alternative promoters and alternative splicing, four or five different proteins may be encoded, in average, by a single gene. Thus, over 200,000 proteins are potentially coded by the set of about 40,000 human genes.

Once synthetized, proteins may udergo post-translational modifications, such as cleavage, glycosylation, phosphorylation and so on, thus increasing the number of different proteins acting at cellular level. The entire set of proteins in a cell or in a tissue is called proteome and the whole network of their meabolic interactions is called metabolome.
->

Preliminary catalogues of genes expressed in the heart, reporting also estimates of the relative expression of each gene are now available.

Mutations in a gene may be pathogenic if the quality or the quantity of its product is affected. Altered function of a protein may cause perturbation in one or more metabolic pathways and it may result in tissue or organ dysfunction. This is the case of most so-called Mendelian disorders, where relationships between gene defects (genotype level) and diseases (phenotype level) may be established. On the contrary, in multifactorial diseases, phenotype is due to a mix of genetic causes (mutations in different genes) and of environmental effects. Mutation in a single gene is a necessary, but not sufficient condition for the development of the disease. Even mutations in several genes may be insufficient to cause the manifestation of the disorder, in the absence of environmental pathogenic factors. Thus, in multifactorial diseases genes contributing to phenotype cannot be considered "disease" genes, but rather "susceptibility" genes.

CHAPTER 3

IDENTIFYING DISEASE GENES IN HUMANS

3.1 Starting with the family

By definition, inherited diseases are expected to run in families. However, due to the peculiarity of the mode of inheritance of each disease, it is possible that a genetically inherited disease is first detected in a family as an isolated case. Often isolated cases are simply due to chance, in regular segregation of a pathogenic mutation in a given family. Let's consider for instance a family in which a dominant mutation with reduced penetrance is inherited (Fig 3.1).

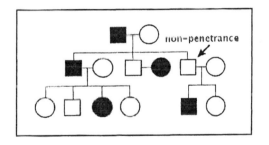

Figure 3.1: Non-penetrance may lead to wrong conclusions about the mode of inheritance of a diseases in a family (see text).

If only the right side of this family tree would be known (i.e. one affected son, born to unaffected parents) the dominant nature of the disease would not be immediately apparent: an affected case born to unaffected parents in one family with no previous history for the disease could be ascribed to homozygosity for an autosomal recessive mutation, inherited from the two heterozygote parents.

If the dominant nature of the disease would be already known, the hypothesis of new mutation could be mistakenly assumed.

In reality, isolated cases due to new mutations (true "sporadics") are rare, although not impossible, especially if a very large gene is involved.

An isolated case manifesting a recessive X-linked disease may appear as a new mutation, especially if the affected male is born to a mother belonging to a small family. It should be remembered that, according to the Haldane's rule, only 1/3 of cases due to X-linked recessive lethal mutations, are due to new mutations. If the disease is sub-lethal, the proportion slightly increases. Therefore, an isolated case affected with one X-linked recessive severe disease (e.g. dilated cardiomyopathy due to dystrophin mutations) would have about 66% probability of being a "false sporadic", having received the pathogenic mutation from previous generations.

Always, when investigating on the possible genetic nature of a disease, particular attention must be paid to family history.

The reconstruction of a family tree requires the assembly of pieces of information collected during interviews with the patient and with additional members of the same family. The person through whom the family was ascertained is called "proband" (or "propositus" if male, "proposita" if female). Proband may not be a patient, but simply a person asking for advise about genetic risk to develop a given disease; for this reason "consultant" may be used instead.

In general, restrospective investigation on a family should involve three generations. The extension of the study to former generations is often useless, for the very good reason that clinical data are usually unavailable for persons diagnosed almost a century ago. On the contrary, restricting the investigation to the last three generations permits to concentrate the effort on a group of persons still alive and who often wish to participate in the study.

In retrospective studies, several problems may be encountered. Affected individual may have died without essential investigations having been done or without autopsy having been performed; some diagnoses may be wrong or firm diagnoses may not have been reached, in spite of accurate clinical investigations.

When starting a retrospective investigation on a family, it is wise to always have in mind that some diagnoses could possibly be wrong or inaccurate.

In case of doubts about clinical features or mode of inheritance, updated information on all inherited disorders known so far is available on-line at the website OMIM (http://www3.ncbi.nlm.nih.gov./omim/).

In order to simplify the record of a family history, a series of symbols (reported in Fig. 3.2) and a standardized procedure are currently used.

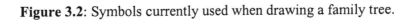

Figure 3.2: Symbols currently used when drawing a family tree.

66

Each horizontal line connecting a male and a female denotes parenthood (if needed, solid line may be used for marriage, dashed line for unmarried couples, although family tree is only intended to show biological relations). A vertical line, descending from this horizontal line and denoting descent, is connected to another horizontal line, to which siblings are individually connected.

Usually, in each couple male (square) is placed on the left side and female (round) on the right. Within each sibship, individuals are ordered from left to right, by order of birth, in declining age. Stillbirths and spontaneous abortions should be recorded, since in some cases they could be associated with genetic defects.

Different generations are indicated by progressive roman numerals (I, II, III, etc), while, within each generation, individuals are indicated by progressive arabic numerals (1, 2, 3, 4, etc), proceeding from left to right, independently from their kindred relations. In this way, each individual may be unequivocally traced within a family tree (Fig.3.3).

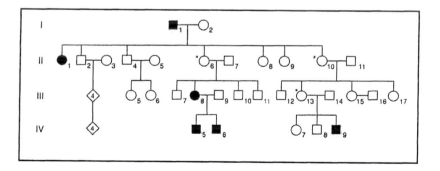

Figure 3.3: A family tree in which numbers of generations (on the left side) and individual numbers are indicated. The disease running in this family is inherited as autosomal dominant trait, with reduced penetrance. Individuals marked by * are non-manifesting obligated carriers of the disease.

In a separate list, the following data should be recorded for each individual:

1) ID number of the person in the family (e.g. II,7)
2) Family name and first name
3) Date and place of birth (and, eventually, date and cause of death)
4) Brief clinical history, including relevant data concerning the specific disease

Once family tree is reconstructed, some individuals may appear to have "a priori" (i.e. genetic) risk of carrying the disease. These persons may be contacted, through the proband, and the possibility of being clinically assessed may be offered to them. For instance, in the family reported in Fig. 3.2, individuals IV,7 and IV,8 appear "at risk", since they could have inherited the pathogenic mutation from their mother, who is the only biological link with other cases manifested in the family. Asymptomatic members at risk (e.g. III,12; III,15 and III,17) should be thoroughly examined, in order to exclude cryptic manifestation of the disease.

As we have seen in section 1.7 of Chapter 1, the investigation in a family may take advantage of analyses on individual DNAs. Each person involved in such a kind of study should sign an appropriate informed consent (see Chapter 6, section 5). In most laboratories and hospitals very strict rules are adopted to protect information on individual DNAs and to code samples stored in DNA banks.

3.2 The positional candidate gene approach

Detecting the gene involved in a given disease is a rather difficult task. However, in some cases simply the inspection of family tree may give useful hints. For instance, a disease with variable manifestations, always transmitted by females to all their offspring, but never inherited from male siblings, would immediately raise the suspect of a mtDNA mutation. On the other hand, the presence of different affections in the same individual, each classified as a mendelian disorder, should suggest the possibility of a deletion involving a rather large chromosomal segment.

A male carrying the deletion in his single X-chromosome, will show a very severe phenotype, due to absence of several genes, but also a person carrying a large deletion in heterozygosity may show a severe and complicated phenotype. If deletion involves a gene-rich chromosomal region, it is highly probable that a deletion would "uncover" deleterious recessive alleles of some genes, thus producing the disease phenotype. This is because each individual is heterozygote for most genes; it has been estimated that every "healthy" person is heterozygote for not less than four lethal mutations.

Sometimes, unusual clinical phenotypes may be due to a micro-deletion which occurred in a chromosome as the breakage point, in an event of translocation. The suspect of a deletion or of a micro-deletion should prompt a cytogenetic investigation, by means of high resolution banding or more sophisticated techniques.

Once detected on a given chromosome, a deletion would immediately locate the genes possibly involved in the disease(s) manifested by the patient.

At the beginning of human molecular genetics this approach, called "deletion mapping", was very helpful in mapping many genes to their respective chromosomal location. Until recently, cytogenetic localization of a disease gene was the first step in a very long, effort- and time-consuming adventure, aiming at establishing a contig of fragments of genomic DNA, covering the entire span of the deleted region. The subsequent search of the wanted disease gene in such contig was usually very frustrating, as looking for a pin in a haystack.

On the contrary, at present, cytogenetic information may be directly used for guiding the search on one of the on-line genomic databases. Updated and ordered series of mapped genes and markers are available at LDB : (http://cedar.genetics.soton.ac.uk/public_html/) or, in alternative, at UDB (http://bioinformatics.weizmann.ac.il/cgi.bin/Udb/). In several cases, the simple inspection of such lists may enable researchers to identify genes which, by their known function, by their tissue-specific expression or by their homology with other genes, could be reasonably taken as candidates for further analysis. This research strategy is called "positional candidate gene approach".

3.3 Linkage analysis in Mendelian diseases

Positional candidate gene approach needs a priori information on approximate location of the gene involved in the genetic disease considered by the investigation.

In the previous section, we have seen that chromosomal deletions and translocations may occasionally help in defining regions harbouring genes involved in the determination of specific clinical phenotypes. However, this possibility is extremely infrequent in reality.

Usually, finding disease genes by positional candidate gene approach mostly relies on linkage studies.

"Linkage" means tendency for some characteristics to be associated in hereditary transmission. We have seen (Chapter 1, section 1.8) that genes carried by different chromosomes undergo independent assortment at meiosis.

Let's consider two genes (A and B), both heterozygous. The heterozygote AA',BB' will have the same chance of transmitting in the same gamete the allele A with the allele B, A with B', A' with B or A' with B'. On the contrary, if gene A would be close to gene B on the same chromosome, it would be highly probable that, being the heterozygote AB/A'B' (A and B on the same chromosome; A' and B' on the homologue) gametes will receive either A and B or A' and B'. Only a crossing over occurring in the chromosomal region between A and B could produce gametes carrying A and B' or A' and B, respectively.

As shown in Fig. 3.4, in a heterozygote for two linked genes there might be two alternative possibilities: 1) mutant alleles (i.e. A' and B') are carried on the same DNA sequence (in this case mutations are said to be carried in "coupling" or "cis"); 2) one mutant allele (e.g. the allele A') is on one chromosome, while the other (B') is on the homologue (in this situation mutations are said to be in "repulsion" or in "trans"). The two described situations correspond to two "linkage phases". The series of alleles at different locations along a single chromosome is called "haplotype", thus haplotypes for the situation of coupling described above would be AB and A'B', while in case of repulsion would be AB' and A'B. A given haplotype will be transmitted unchanged through generations, unless modified by recombination.

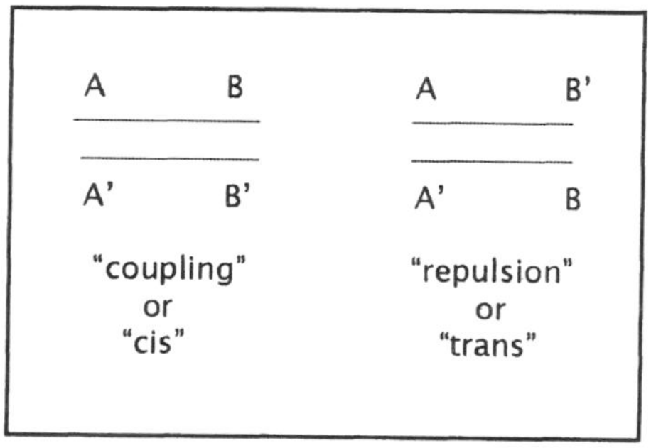

Figure 3.4: Linkage phases. The double heterozygote AA'BB' may carry mutant alleles either in "cis" or in "trans". Different haplotypes are indicated. Thus, a heterozygote AA'BB' may be either AB/A'B' or AB'/A'B.

The greater the physical distance between A and B, greater will be the probability of occurrence of a crossing-over. Therefore, recombination frequency, which depends on the rate of crossing-overs, is roughly proportional to the distance between two selected points (loci) on a given chromosome. "Locus" is the place of a given gene or of a given marker, along a specific chromosome.

If two genes are close by , they are said to be " tightly linked". Their respective alleles will tend to be always transmitted "in linkage" (e.g. A with B and A' with B'). The tightness of linkage between two loci can be measured in "units of recombination". One recombination unit, called centiMorgan (cM), corresponds to 1% recombination and to a real length of about 1 Mb (1 million nucleotides) on the chromosomal DNA. The value of recombination fraction is indicated by the symbol ϑ (theta).

The method for detecting and estimating linkage in humans was developed by N.E. Morton in 1955, based on the computation of "lod scores".

"Lod score" (symbolized by Z) is literally the log of the odds (Log of the ODds) in favour of the hypothesis of linkage of a genetic marker (e.g. a given polymorphic DNA marker) to a given phenotype (e.g. a given disease), as opposed to random segregation ("non-linkage") which occurs when the two considered loci are far apart or in different chromosomes.

Given a family in which two genetically inherited characteristics (e.g., as we said, affection status and typing for a specific marker) can be precisely determined, and selected a given value of theta (e.g. $\vartheta = 0$ for complete lingage) probability is calculated that the observed segregation of phenotypes is due to linkage between the two loci. A second probability value is computed, assuming the alternative hypothesis, i.e. that the two considered loci are unlinked.

The lod score value, corresponding to the log of the ratio between the first and the second probability value, will tell us if the hypothesis of linkage is acceptable.

$$\text{Lod score} (Z) = \log \frac{\text{Conditional probability (linkage)}}{\text{Conditional probability (independence)}}$$

Z values over +3 are in favour of linkage; values over +6 point at highly significant evidence of linkage, while Z values less than –2 exclude the existence of linkage between the considered loci. Z values between –2 and +3 are inconclusive.

The calculation of the Z value must be performed for different values of theta (0.0, 0.05, 0.10, 0.20, 0.30, 0.40). Therefore, in the past computation of lod scores was a very laborious and tedious work. Fortunately, in 1984 Lathrop and Lalouel produced a software (LINKAGE) for automatic calculation of lod scores. The program, originally written in Pascal, is still widely used and it is available also at the HGMP (Human Genome Mapping Project) server (http:// www.hgmp.mrc.ac.uk/). Input of data requires some care and time, but results may be obtained, at most, in a few minutes.

A typical table of lod scores is reported in Tab. 3.1.

M	Recombination fraction								
	0.00	0.01	0.05	0.10	0.20	0.30	0.40	θmax	zmax
A	-0.52	1.69	2.15	2.13	1.75	1.18	0.52	0.05	2.15
B	3.37	3.30	3.04	2.71	1.99	1.20	0.42	0.00	3.37
C	3.73	3.67	3.41	3.07	2.34	1.54	0.67	0.00	3.73
D	3.69	3.62	3.37	3.03	2.31	1.52	0.67	0.00	3.69
E	3.06	3.00	2.78	2.50	1.89	1.22	0.51	0.00	3.06
F	-2.23	-1.53	-0.36	0.07	0.33	0.32	0.18	0.20	0.33

Table 3.1: A lod score table, in which values of Z corresponding to different thetas are reported for five different polymorphic DNA markers (M). Markers are aligned along a given chromosomal region. In this case, some markers show values of Z above the threshold of significance (+3), thus suggesting linkage with the disease locus. The region where the unknown gene should be searched is probably included between markers A and F (by courtesy of Dr. A. Rampazzo)

Usually values of Z are calculated for theta values corresponding respectively to 0.0, 0.1, 0.2, 0.3 and 0.4. However, by LINKAGE software it is possible to calculate Z for any pre-selected value of theta. The series of five values corresponding respectively to the different hypotheses of linkage provides sufficiently precise information about linkage relationships. Z value corresponding to theta=0.5 is not shown, since it corresponds to the null hypothesis (i.e. independent segregation of the considered loci).

Each family is composed of two original parents, their offspring and descendants, plus respective mates and sibs. Each individual born to a couple is the product of paternal and maternal gametes, produced by meiosis. Therefore, when analyzing the offspring of a given couple, in reality we are looking at the products of their meioses.

The possibility of detecting recombinations in the haplotypes depends on the "informativity" of paternal and maternal meiosis. If an individual is heterozygote at two loci (AA'BB') and the phase is known (e.g AB/A'B'), by examining the genotype of the offspring it would be possible to detect recombinations. However, if the individual is homozygote in one locus (AABB') it would be impossible to detect a recombination which eventually occurred between locus A and locus B, since allele A in one chromosome is indistinguishable from the allele A of the homologous chromosome. In this case meiose would be uninformative for locus A, informative for locus B, but not informative on the whole.

Two different situations in which a meiose is uninformative are shown in Fig. 3.5. The gene is assumed to be transmitted linked to the marker A and its mutation is assumed to have dominant effect.

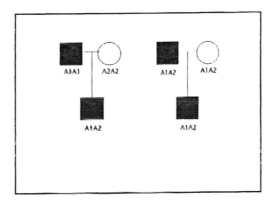

Figure 3.5: Two cases of uniformative meioses (see text for explanation)

On the left side, paternal meiose is uninformative because it would be impossible to establish which paternal homologue was transmitted to the affected son (both homologues are "marked" by an allele A1). On the right, paternal meiosis is potentially informative, but the mother shows heterozygosity for the same alleles. Again, it would be impossible to understand which paternal homologue transmitted the disease to the son. The situation would be different if the mother was, for instance, A3A4 and the son A1A4.

Situations of non-informativity of some meioses are not infrequent in families. Thus, actual lod scores may result much lower than expected by assuming that all meioses were informative.

In linkage analysis, the possibility of obtaining significant lod scores depends on the number of informative meioses. In practice, not less than 15 informative meioses are needed in three generations, to obtain a Z value around +3.

In most cases, families showing the presence of a genetic disease are limited in size (i.e. from 10 to 20 individuals in three generations). Due to the non-informativity of some meioses and to non-availability of some samples (because of death or because refusal to give a blood sample for DNA analyses), it is hard to obtain significant evidence of linkage. However, due to property of logarithms, Z values obtained in unrelated families showing the same disease and tested for the same markers may be added, to produce a "collective" value of Z, which, if significantly positive, would prove linkage.

This procedure may be jeopardized by genetic heterogeneity, i.e. by existence of families showing diseases with identical or very similar clinical phenotype, but of different genetic origin. In cardiomyopathies, genetic heterogeneity seems to be the rule rather than exception: several genetically different forms were described so far in hypetrophic cardiomyopathy, in dilated cardiomyopathy and in arrhythmogenic right ventricular cardiomyopathy (see Chapter 4).

Genetic heterogeneity should always be suspected, because it is a very common phenomenon. Therefore, when planning a linkage study, it is better to concentrate efforts in obtaining data from a single and relatively large family, rather than collecting information on a large number of nuclear families.

In general, once one family tree is reconstructed, it is possible to obtain by simulation the corresponding maximum potential value of Z, by using the program S-LINK of the LINKAGE package: if Z would be just above +3, the risk of a failure is very high.

The search for linkage in human families affected with a dominant mendelian disorder is currently performed by a procedure called "genome-wide search" or "genome scan".

The principle is simple: given hundreds DNA markers regularly spaced along the entire human genome, linkage with the disease locus is tested for each of them and lod score is computed. Significant lod scores would indicate the chromosomal region where the disease gene is located.

Linkage mapping sets are available in commerce, consisting of fluorescently labeled PCR primer pairs, selected to amplify two-base pair repeat microsatellites previously mapped to precise locations of genomic DNA.

The most widely used is the ABI PRISM Linkage Mapping Set, available in two densities of markers (5 cM and 10 cM resolution). PCR amplification conditions are standardized and markers are arranged in panels according to the type of the fluorescent dye and the size of the amplification product, in order to enable simultaneous analysis of dozen of PCR products, separated by electrophoresis in a DNA automatic sequencer

Usually, in each lane, amplicons corresponding to a dozen of markers are separated, but, by expoiting differences in molecular size and in fluorescent dye, up to twenty markers can be analyzed in a single run. A typical output, corresponding to amplicons obtained in different individual DNAs for a single DNA marker and separated by an automated DNA sequencer, is shown in Fig. 3.6.

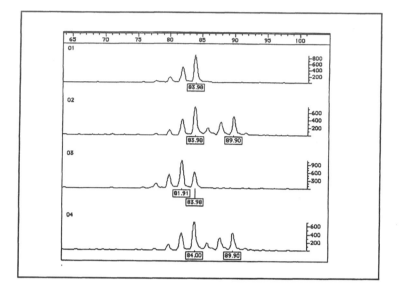

Figure 3.6: Electrophoretic separation of PCR amplicons by an automatic DNA sequencer. Each lane correspond to the separation of amplification products obtained from genomic DNA of a single individual by PCR primers corresponding to a given microsatellite DNA marker. Lane 01: homozygous genotype; lanes 02 and 04: heterozygotes for the same alleles; lane 03: heterozygote for a different allele. Only portion of the lane corresponding to the selected marker is shown. (by courtesy of Dr. S. Malacrida)

Given a family with 30 members, a genome scan using 700 DNA markers would imply 21,000 individual PCR reactions and the visual inspection of the corresponding results. Specific software (GENESCAN, GENOTYPER, LINKAGE DESIGNER, LINKAGE, LINKAGE REPORTER) are used for the different steps of the analysis. The final result will be exclusion of linkage for a large number of markers (entire chromosomes might result excluded) and evidence of linkage of the disease with some markers. However, non-informativity of some markers may produce false negative results, thus forcing the researcher to perform a new run of linkage analysis on non-excluded chromosomal regions, by using additional markers.

In spite of partial automatization, genome scan is time- and effort-consuming: one experieced person should spend about 4 months of work to complete a genome-wide search in a family.

Recently, novel DNA-chip technology, in conjunction with genetic map of SNPs, was introduced. Commercial DNA chips are available, where over 1,400 SNP markers may be interrogated, thus providing about 1,200-1,300 SNP genotypes per DNA sample.

By each chip, the genotype of a single individual can be obtained. Therefore, 30 chips would be needed for performing a linkage study in a family with 30 members. This technology is still rather expensive, however it is gaining popularity, since it greatly reduces time and laboratory work, with no apparent decrease in efficiency.

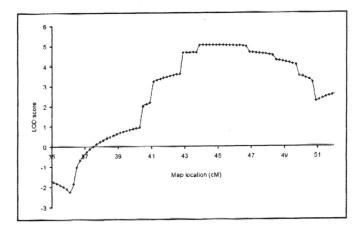

Figure 3.7: Graphical output of a multipoint linkage analysis. Lod scores peak in correspondence of the probable location of the disease gene, within the segment where ordered DNA markers are located on the x axis (by courtesy of Dr. A. Vettori).

Once significant evidence of linkage would be obtained for a given chromosomal region, additional two-point lod scores should be obtained for additional polymorphic DNA markers mapped to the region and reported in

78

Human Genome Browser, in order to restrict the "critical region", i.e. the segment of genomic DNA harbouring the searched disease gene.

Lod score data obtained by this additional study are used for performing a "multipoint linkage analysis". The program LINKMAP of the package LINKAGE calculates lod scores for the placement of the disease locus in a given grid of ordered markers. The graphical representation of the results of a multipoint linkage analysis is reported in Fig. 3.7. The larger the number of closely spaced markers in the critical region, the sharper will be the localization of the disease gene.

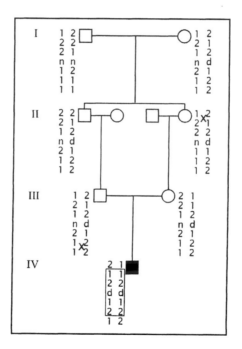

Figure 3.8: Principle of "homozygosity mapping". Mutant alleles found in homozygosity (dd) in the affected individual may be traced back to one ancestor (maternal great-grand mother). The ancestral haplotype is fully conserved for markers closely linked to the disease locus, while recombinations (X) occurred distally (d= disease allele, n= normal allele). For each individual in the family tree, genotypes for each of six DNA markers loci are show. Markers are in the same order as they are on the chromosome.

When dealing with autosomal recessive diseases, the approach for detecting linkage in families is to some extent simplified by the adoption of a method described by Lander and Botstein in 1987.

Individuals homozygous for a recessive pathogenic mutation often occur in the offspring of marriages between blood relatives (e.g. first-cousins) or between persons belonging to the same isolated and inbred population. Actually, it is highly probable that in such instances the affected individual would have inherited from the same ancestor the two mutant alleles, one from the paternal side and the other from the maternal side. He can be defined "homozygous by descent" (Fig. 3.8).

Because of the small number of generations (i.e. of meioses) intervened between the ancestor and the affected individual, the probability that a crossing over would have occurred in close proximity of the disease gene is very low. Therefore, it is expected that the affected individual is homozygous as well for a series of DNA markers, contiguous to the disease locus.

Genotyping for DNA markers is performed as in wide-genome search and by using the same panels of markers, but in this case only DNAs of affected individuals are analyzed.

In general, analysis of genotypes of 700-800 DNA markers in a dozen of individuals affected with the same recessive disease would suffice to provide evidence of linkage, if any, between disease locus and flanking markers. However, as in dominant diseases, the possible confounding effect of genetic heterogeneity must always be taken into consideration.

3.4 Linkage analysis in multifactorial diseases

As shown in Section 3.3, in monogenic diseases linkage analysis is performed on specific assumptions about mode of inheritance, number of alleles, penetrance, etc.

When dealing with multifactorial diseases (see Chapter 2, section 2.9), the situation is complicated by absence of clear information about dominance or recessivity of mutations in genes contributing to genetic determination of liability. Actually, mutations in some genes involved in a given disease, may act as dominants, while mutations in other genes might behave as recessives. Therefore, standard linkage analysis (also called "parametric linkage analysis" or "model-based linkage analysis" cannot be applied. Instead, non-parametric ("model-free") methods of linkage analysis have been developed for the purpose, which rely only on the simple assumption that two affected relatives should share alleles predisposing to disease.

"Affected sibpair" method, developed by Weeks and Lange in 1992, considers only siblings concordant for the manifestation of a given disease.

As shown in Fig. 3.9, two concordant sibs born to a couple of heterozygotes in a single gene may have four different genotypes (A1A3, A1A4,A2A3,A2A4). As shown in the little table within the figure, they would inherit the same two alleles with 25% probability, one allele in common with 50% probability and no allele in common with 25% probability.

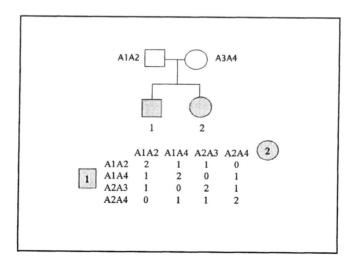

Figure 3.9: Principle of the "affected sibpair" method (see text for explanation). In the lower part of the figure, the possible combinations of pairs with given genotypes are reported.

If predisposition to a given disease would be due to mutations in a specific gene, since this gene would be in linkage with its flanking markers, affected siblings should share marker alleles above expected 50% .

In order to prove a significant deviation from the expectation, a large number of sib pairs is needed. For instance, to detect an allele-sharing ratio of 60% , about 200 pairs of sibs would be required.

In the "highly discordant sibpair" method, highly discordant sibs are assumed to show no allele-sharing at the loci involved in the determination of the considered trait. Therefore, genome scan is performed to find those chromosomal regions where alleles are shared among sibs less frequently than expected.

TDT (Transmission Disequilibrium Test) was developed by Spielman et al. (1993). Families with one or more affected sibs are considered, in which one parent should show heterozygosity for a given allele of the marker locus, suspected to be linked to the disease allele. The theoretical ground of this test is that the frequency of the selected allele marker among affected sibs would be expectedly higher, if this allele is really linked to the disease allele. Let $\underline{a}$ be the frequency by which the heterozygote parent transmits the given marker allele (e.g.A') to the affected sibs, and $\underline{b}$ the frequency by which the other marker allele (e.g. A") is transmitted. A chi-square test with one degree of freedom is performed:

$$\text{TDT chi-square (1 d.f)} = (a-b)^2/(a+b)$$

Significant chi-square values would indicate that allele marker A' and disease allele are preferably transmitted associated. This test is reliable only if the sample of families is large.

A different method of "disease association" study, is finding whether a particular allele in a marker locus shows increased frequency among affected individuals rather than among unaffected controls. The strength of the association is expressed by "odds ratio":

$$odds\ ratio = \text{ad/bc}$$

where $\underline{a}$ is the number of patients carrying a given allele, $\underline{b}$ the number of controls showing such allele, $\underline{c}$ and $\underline{d}$ the number of patients and, respectively, of controls not carrying the allele. Odds ratio equals 1 when the frequency is the same in patients and in controls.

In all these studies, the number of subjects to be analyzed by genome scan is very high. For this reason, association studies are difficult to perform, but a progress in this field is ahead. A genetic map of SNPs, in conjunction with new DNA-chip technology would allow in future efficient screening of the entire human genome of large number of persons affected with common diseases, thus providing a huge potential for locating susceptibility genes for multifactorial diseases. For the moment, different studies are in progress, based on the genotyping of very large samples of human populations, by using about 2,000 SNPs. The aim of these studies is to establish clear relationships between individual clinical data concerning common diseases and individual genotype data.

Paradoxically, in these studies genotyping is far less problematic than phenotyping. Actually, while experimental variability may be minimized by selection of appropriate technology and experimental design, variability in diagnoses would still remain very high, because a large population sample implies a large number of doctors involved in clinical diagnoses.

This variability would further increase if the study would be conducted on very large population samples, as required by this kind of investigations. In a large geographical area differences are expected in hospital standards and in ethnical and social composition of the population.

Fig. 3.10 illustrates relationships between different approaches for searching genes involved in multifactorial diseases. Novel candidate loci may derive from studies on animal models (e.g. rat model of hypertension): if one gene presumably involved in the considered disease would be located on the genetic map of the animal, it could be possible to detect the corresponding candidate locus on the human genetic map, by exploiting methods of comparative genomics.

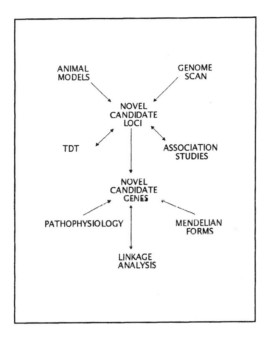

Figure 3.10: Different approaches for searching genes involved in multifactorial diseases (see text for explanation).

This approach is greatly facilitated if the animal model is mouse, since the DNA sequence of the entire genome of this animal has been recently released.

On the other hand, candidate loci may be identified by genome scanning applied to human sibpairs, by association studies and by TDT (Transmission Disequilibrium Test).

If a putative locus would be detected by applying one method, an independent study performed by a different method should give concordant results. Unfortunately, this is not always the case.

Finally, candidate genes may be obtained by inspection of the critical region (positional approach), by analogy with genes known to be involved in mendelian disorders phenotypically similar to the disease under study (comparative approach), or by understanding molecular pathogenesis of the disease (pathophysiological approach).

As recently pointed out (Swyngedauw, 2002), candidate gene method requires: a) functional candidate genes and functional mutations fully documented by animal experiments; b) high statistical power (N>200-400; p<0.01); c) clear definition of phenotype, by randomly selected homogeneous cohorts of patients; d) possibly, information on the heritability of the trait and on frequency in the population.

In conclusion, in spite of their apparent simplicity, association studies are particularly difficult to perform. A recent study critically reviewed a large series of association studies. Six hundred associations between common gene variants and diseases were reported; however only 166 putative associations were studied three or more times and only 6 have been consistently replicated (Hirschhorn, 2002).

3.5 Detecting pathogenic mutations

The problem of detecting DNA mutations is of paramount importance both in research (finding genes involved in inherited diseases) and in practice (attempting to detect carriers of pathogenic mutations in families).

The most efficient method for detecting point mutations is obviously DNA sequencing. Automated DNA sequencers, based on capillary electrophoresis technology, are very efficient and precise. They produce digital output files which are automatically converted into pictures, called "chromatograms", since they are diagrams in colours (no relation with "chromatography"!).

In these pictures, the reading of each band is represented by a peak (intensity of recorded fluorescence); all peaks corresponding to a given nucleotide type have the same colour (e.g. green for adenine, red for thymine, blue for cytosine, black for guanine). The series of coloured peaks corresponds to the series of nucleotides in the analyzed DNA sequence. A single base change may be clearly detected, as shown in Fig. 3.11.

Automated DNA sequencers are standard equipment in many laboratories and price per sequence is reasonable. Therefore, mutation screening by sequencing is gaining more and more popularity. However, identification of mutations in very large genes remains expensive, especially for diagnostic purposes. A mutation screening of the entire RyR2 gene (105 exons!) would cost not less than 1,300 $ per patient.

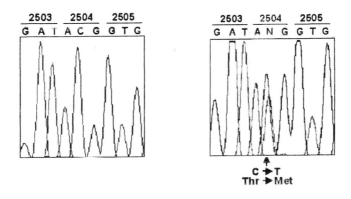

Figure 3.11: Output of DNA sequencing. The notation N in the sequence on top of the figure on the right side means that the automated DNA sequencer couldn't automatically assign a nucleotide to that position. In fact, visual inspection reveals that in such position there are two peaks. By comparison with the sequence of a control DNA (on the left side), it is possible to establish that a mutation has occurred and that the type of change was C->T. A double peak denotes heterozygosity for the mutation (by courtesy of Dr. A. Bagattin).

An advantage of direct DNA sequencing is that primers for PCR amplification are usually designed in intronic sequences flanking each exon; therefore, eventual splice site mutations may be detected as well. On the contrary, direct sequencing is unable to detect single- or multiple-exon deletions, since sequence of a normal DNA strand in double dose would be identical to that of a normal DNA in single dose. For detection of intragenic deletions or duplications, digestion with restriction enzymes and Southern blot should be used (see later, this Chapter).

Mutation screening by direct sequencing may be performed on cDNA, instead that on genomic DNA. In this case, the sample should derive from the diseased tissue, because of possible differential expression of the considered gene.

In the last two decades, when DNA sequencing was considered still unpractical, a series of alternative laboratory methods have been proposed. Most of them are based on the principle that a nucleotide change in a DNA sequence may be indirectly detected through the formation of heteroduplexes.

Let's consider a nucleotide change in an exon of a given gene and an individual heterozygote for such mutation. If we amplify by PCR that exon, among amplification products we will find both mutant and normal amplicons. At this point, if the mixture of amplicons is heated to denaturation and then cooled gradually, re-naturation will produce three species of double-stranded DNA molecules: normal-normal and mutant-mutant homoduplexes, plus normal-mutant heteroduplexes.(Fig. 3.12)

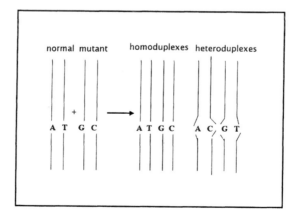

Figure 3.12: Formation of heteroduplexes when two double strands of DNA differing by one nucleotide are denatured and re-natured.

Heteroduplexes will have, in correspondence of the mutated nucleotide, a small zone of imperfect pairing ("mismatch"). This peculiarity of heteroduplexes may be conveniently exploited to detect the presence of a unknown mutation, since mismatches offer the possibility of differentiating homoduplexes from heteroduplexes.

A number of laboratory methods have been developed, based on this principle.

Heteroduplex mismatch may be detected by chemical or by enzymatic cleavage. If cleavage is followed by electrophoretic separation, the presence of a mutation will be inferred if abnormal, small-size products, would be observed. Chemical cleavage is a high sensitive method, but it it is experimentally difficult   and it requires handling toxic chemicals (hydroxylamine and osmium tetroxide). For this reason this method never encountered the favour of the laboratory people. On the other hand, enzymatic cleavage never showed to produce high quality results.

Heteroduplexes have different electrophoretic mobility than homoduplexes. Therefore, mobility shifts detected in polyacrylamide gel electrophoresis would indicate the presence of heteroduplexes. This method is very simple and cheap, but it works only with DNA sequences shorter than 200 nt and its sensitivity is limited, even using special gel matrices (e.g. Hydrolink or MDE).

DGGE (Denaturing Gradient Gel Electrophoresis) is based on the principle that heteroduplexes have abnormal profiles of denaturation and that the mobility of DNA molecule changes when denaturation occurs. Therefore, in a denaturing gradient gel, mobility shift of heteroduplexed will be amplified. DGGE requires a special thermally controlled equipment for electrophoresis and special PCR primers, carrying a 5' poly-GC sequence ("GC clamp"). After optimization, which requires time and effort, DGGE may reach high sensitivity.

The most popular among "simple methods" for mutation detection is SSCP (Single Strand Conformation Polymorphism) (Fig. 3.13).

SSCP relies on the property of single-stranded DNA filaments to form in solution three-dimensional folded structures, stabilized by base-pairing hydrogen bonds. Mutant DNA may form three-dimensional structures different from normal. Since electrophoretic mobility of single-stranded DNA molecules in a non-denaturing polyacrylamide gel would depend on the conformation of the three-dimensional structure, we may expect to observe a "polymorphism", i.e. a difference, in electrophoretic mobility between normal and mutant molecules.

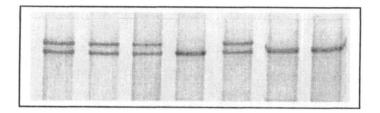

Figure 3.13: SSCP. Silver-stained polyacrylamide gel clearly shows two-banded patterns, corresponding to the presence of both normal and mutant conformations; single bands correspond to normals (by courtesy of Dr. G. Beffagna).

In SSCP, PCR amplification products are denatured and loaded on a non-denaturing gel. After electrophoresis, gel is silver-stained. Abnormal mobility shifts would denounce the presence of a mutation.

SSCP sensitivity is optimal (up to 80%) for fragments about 200 nt in length, but it decreases with increasing size of the amplification products.

The popularity of the method is due to the very favourable combination of very low cost, simplicity of the protocol and, last but not least, good sensitivity.

A novel method, which recently gained the favour of laboratories, is named DHPLC (or dHPLC = Denaturing High Pressure Liquid Chromatography), based on the principle that DNA molecules may be separated by liquid chromatography, according to their size.

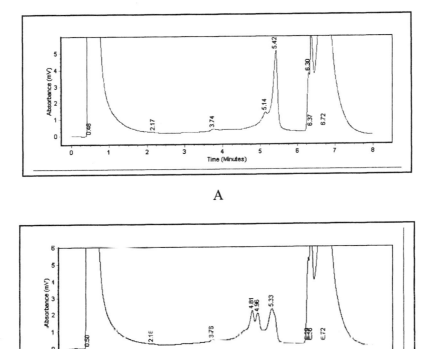

A

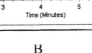

B

Figure 3.14: Elution patterns obtained in DHPLC analysis of PCR amplicons corresponding to exon of exon 3 of RYR2 gene. A: elution of a normal exon; B: elution of a mutated exon. In correspondence of retention time between 5 and 6 minutes, a novel peak pattern can be clearly noticed, due to a point mutation (by courtesy of Dr. A. Bagattin).

After having been subjected to denaturation and re-naturation, DNA samples are placed in a DPLC apparatus, where analysis is performed at a temperature sufficient to partially denature heteroduplexes. Since partial denaturation reduces the double-stranded portion of the DNA molecule, partially denatured molecules (heteroduplexes) will be eluted before homoduplexes. Therefore, in case of mutation, a novel peak of elution will appear, before the peak corresponding to homoduplexes (Fig. 3.14). The quality of the separation strongly depends on the elution conditions.

In the near future, technology of DNA chips will probably make obsolete most of the present methods. Oligonucleotide arrays and minisequencing DNA chips are ahead.

Some large genes are prone to intragenic deletions or duplications, spanning several Kb. In these cases, the above described methods, devised for detecting "point" mutations, are useless.

Although protocols for semi-quantitative PCR amplification are available for the purpose, old-fashioned Southern blot is still the most efficient method for detecting intragenic deletions and duplications.

Genomic DNAs from samples and from controls are digested by a restriction enzyme (usually HindIII). The mixture of fragments obtained by this digestion is separated on horizontal agarose gel electrophoresis and resulting bands are transferred to a nylon membrane by Southern blotting. Then, cDNA probes obtained from the selected gene are radioactively labelled and hybridized to nylon membrane.

After autoradiography, the pattern of bands observed in samples is compared to that of controls. Abnormal bands would denounce, according to their number and electrophoretic mobility, the presence of deletions or of duplications.

Southern blot is also used to detect the presence of triplet nucleotide expansions.

3.6 Establishing the pathogenic role of specific mutations

In previous sections we considered the strategy for identifying disease loci and we said that once a locus would be identified, a number of candidate genes for such disease could be obtained by bioinformatic search on Human Genome Browser.

Mutation screening methods are applied to such candidate genes, in order to find if DNA obtained from affected persons (belonging to a family in which the disease is transmitted linked to the given locus) carries a mutation.

In order to prove that one candidate gene is indeed the gene involved in the determination of the disease, its mutation should explain the manifestation of the disease.

Detecting a mutation in a candidate gene is an exciting result, but often it is not enough to prove that the gene is really involved in the determination of the disease.

While a novel stop codon would clearly point at a causative mutation, a missense mutation could simply correspond to a non-pathogenic DNA polymorphism. Therefore, this possibility should be ruled out. To this purpose, the presence of the detected mutation must be checked in a series of 300-500 DNAs from healthy and unrelated controls, taken from the population in which the mutation was detected.

Negative findings after screening 500 individuals (i.e. 1,000 chromosomes) would mean that the frequency of the mutant allele is possibly less than 1/1000. Thus, the hypothesis of having detected a rare non pathogenic variant would appear improbable, although it couldn't be totally dismissed.

However, if this mutation would produce an aminoacid change significantly altering the shape of the alpha helix or the polarity of a residue, the hypothesis of a functional consequence of the mutation would gain credit.

Comparing the aminoacid sequence of the human protein coded by the gene with sequences of proteins coded by orthologous genes (i.e the same gene in different animal species) may be very helpful, since mutations in highly conserved domains usually alter protein function.

After having detected one supposedly pathogenic mutation, a series of further questions should be answered:

1) In which tissues is the gene expressed and at which level?
2) What is the normal function of the gene?

92

3) What could be the effect of a mutation?

4) What could be, in particular, the effect of the detected mutation?

Experimental approach may be easy in some cases, very difficult in others. For instance, differential expression in human tissues may be easily assessed by PCR amplification on cDNAs from different tissues, by using commercial kits, as shown in Fig. 3.15.

On the contrary, it could be rather difficult to understand what is the normal function of the gene or what could be the effect of its mutation, in absence of relevant biochemical information. Some hints can be obtained by bioinformatic analysis of the protein sequence, by analyzing the nature of detectable protein domains and by comparing them with similar domains already described and characterized in other organisms.

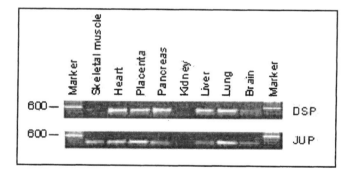

Figure 3.15: Assessment of gene expression in different human tissues. In this case the expression of plakoglobin gene (involved in Naxos disease) and of desmoplakin gene (involved in Carvajal syndrome, Naxos-like disease) are compared. Both genes appear expressed in heart. Desmoplakin shows no expression in skeletal muscle (by courtesy of Dr. A. Rampazzo).

Functional studies are effort- and time-consuming, but they are the only way to prove the effect of mutation at biochemical level. Production of an animal model, by artificial mutation of the orthologous gene, may appear as a shortcut, but in reality this work is not simple at all. Gene "knock-out" in mouse (artificial production of a defective mutant, in single or double dosage, see Chapter 4, section 5) may prove that a given mutation produces a phenotypic change.

However, sometimes the phenotype corresponding to a given gene defect in mice is different from the human disease phenotype, because of differences in functional relationships between the corresponding protein products at biochemical level, or because differences in the genetic background (laboratory mice are usually from inbred strains, while humans are heterozygous at most loci).

3.7 Establishing genotype-phenotype correlations

Paradoxically, the most important contribution to the understanding of molecular genetics of inherited diseases comes not from DNA studies, but from clinical studies.

Linkage study provides information about the locus involved and enables to select groups of families in which the disease is transmitted linked to the same DNA markers, i.e. likely to to mutations of the same gene.

This information alone is very valuable for a preliminary study at phenotype level. All patients with affections belonging to the same linkage group are expected to share the same phenotypic traits of the disease, like symptoms or response to a specific treatment. Inter-familial variability would suggest the possibility that different mutations of the same gene might produce different effects, or it could point at "family factors" due to common environment , e.g. diet or infections.

On the other hand, intra-familial variability would suggest the role of additional genes in shaping the clinical phenotype, or the role of selective environmental factors. For instance, in some cardiomyopathies, participation of some family members in competitive sport in the teen age could produce a large variability in clinical phenotypes among adults of the same family.

Once a gene mutation is detected and characterized in a family, important information may be obtained on the role of additional genes or of environmental factors, by comparing clinical presentations among relatives sharing the same mutation,.

In all these instances the role of the Clinician is fundamental for further progress of our knowledge. It should be remember that, in oder to enable proper comparisons and statistical treatment of data, observations should be always transformed in numerical parameters, i.e. in measurements.

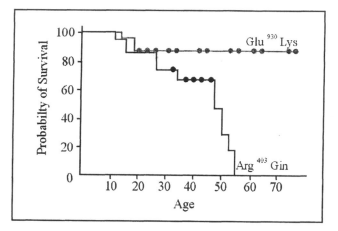

Figure 3.16 : Survival curves in two families affected with hypertrophic cardiomyopathy, due to two different mutations of gene coding for beta-myosin heavy chain. (from Marian, modified)

Genotype-phenotype correlations may be obtained for different mutations of the same gene. As shown by Fig. 3.16, one mutation may be associated with a relatively benign prognosis, while the other may produce a more severe affection and higher risk of sudden death.

Evaluation and re-evaluation of clinical data in the light of the identification of gene mutations underlying clinical phenotypes is one of the most promising fields of clinical cardiology. Knowing the gene involved in a specific mendelian disease and the particular mutation running in a given family affected with that disease would enable to firmly establish the intrinsic genetic risk of each individual, before manifestation of any clinical symptom.

This would allow to adopt early preventive measures and timely setting of proper treatment.

Moreover, as shown in Fig. 3.16, knowledge of the consequence of given mutations might help in establishing prognosis.

SUMMARY After the sequencing of human DNA was completed, bioinformatic analysis succeeded in identifying almost all human genes. However, linking mutations of each gene to a genetic disease is still progressing with some difficulty.

Identification of a gene involved in determination of a Mendelian disorder usually requires preliminary chromosomal localization of its locus, i.e. the region including the gene. For such a purpose, linkage analysis is usually applied to three-generation families with a sufficient number of sibs. The success of linkage analysis is strictly dependent on clear definition of disease phenotype, which enables dicrimination between "affected" and non-affected" individuals. In a genome scan, linkage analysis involves testing each individual with 700 DNA polymorphic markers, which location is already established along human chromosomes. Linkage analysis in multifactorial diseases is performed by non-parametric methods, aiming at establishing if a given marker variant is inherited significantly associated with the disease in a large cohort of sibs. This kind of study is complicated by the fact that not always "predisposing" genotypes correspond to diseased phenotype and that genetic heterogeneity is possible.

A gene may be considered as a candidate because it is located within the "critical" chromosomal region, because the function of its product is related to the defect, or for both reasons (positional and functional candidate approach). In order to prove that a candidate gene is indeed involved in the determination of the disease, it is necessary to prove that mutations of such gene are pathogenic.   >

The most simple approach is to screen for mutations the coding sequences of the gene, by using direct DNA sequencing or DHPLC analysis

These methods are suitable for detecting single nucleic acid substitutions, deletions or duplications On the contrary, for detection of intragenic deletions or duplications of large segments of DNA, different methods must be applied. Nonsense mutations, i.e. nucleotide substitutions generating a stop codon, and gross gene alterations may be immediately suspected to be pathogenic, while in case of missense mutations, i.e. nucleotide substitutions producing an aminoacid change in the coded protein, the demonstration of their pathogenicity may be more problematic.

CHAPTER 4

INHERITED STRUCTURAL AND FUNCTIONAL DEFECTS OF MYOCARDIUM

4.1 Cardiomyopathies

Cardiomyopathies are diseases of myocardium, associated with cardiac dysfunction. They are the most common cause of heart failure in humans; some of them are associated with sudden juvenile death.

By gross morphological characteristics, cardiomyopathies may be classified into four groups: Dilative cardiomyopathies, Hypertrophic cardiomyopathies, Arrhythmogenic right ventricular cardiomyopathies and Restrictive cardiomyopathies. Each group includes a rather heterogeneous series of diseases, mostly genetic in origin. Wolfang (2001) and Towbin (2002) provided comprehensive reviews on this subject.

The role of gene mutations in human cardiomyopathies is increasingly recognized. In the last few years several genes involved in such diseases have been identified and many causative mutations have been described.

In the following account it was selected to provide for each disease the ID number corresponding to the record in OMIM. This should facilitate the reader to permanently access detailed and updated information on clinical and genetical aspects of a given disorder. For the same reason, acronyms used in this text are according to OMIM nomenclature (e.g CMH for Hypertrophic Cardiomyopathy, rather than HCM or FHCM).

It should be remembered that OMIM is a catalogue, in which classification is grounded on main clinical features. Therefore, it provides little help in fine differential diagnosis at clinical level. On the contrary, its permanent collection of data on genes, mutations and clinical phenotypes provides an invaluable tool for guiding in molecular genetic investigation and in differential diagnosis based on DNA analysis.

Possibly, in the near future diseases will be grouped by genotypes, rather than by phenotypes. In front of possible change in classification and nomenclature, OMIM numbers will represent a firm reference.

Hypertrophic cardiomyopathy (CMH=CardioMyopathy, Hypetrophic, also indicated by the acronym HCM=Hypetrophic CardioMyopathy) is possibly the main cause of cardiac sudden death among young adults and athletes. The prevalence rate of CMH is not yet firmly established. However, in a large cohort of apparently healthy young individuals selected from a community-based population, echocardiographic evaluation revealed a prevalence of about 0.2% (Maron, 1997).

Most commonly, CMH is manifested before age 25. A significant proportion of affected persons develop congestive heart failure.

Main feature of CMH is thickness of intraventricular septum and of left ventricular posterior wall.

CMH appears as a familial disease in about 50% of cases. The fraction of *de novo* mutations among isolated cases is still unknown. Like CMD, hypertrophic cardiomyopathy shows large genetic heterogeneity. Nine different forms of CMH are listed in OMIM. In seven of them involved genes are known. Mutations causing CMH were identified so far in additional nuclear genes and in mtDNA (Tab. 4.1). Molecular genetic investigation on CMH started in 1989, when a linkage study (lod score 9.37 at theta 0) mapped a CMH locus to chromosome 14 (14q11-q12). Because myosin heavy chain genes (MYH6 and MYH7) were mapped to the same chromosomal region, such genes were immediately considered as candidate genes.

Table 4.1: Genetic heterogeneity in CMHs. (I: mode of inheritance; AD: autosomal dominant; AR: autosomal recessive; XL: X-linked; mt: carried by mitochondrial DNA)

Type	Locus	I	Gene	OMIM
CMH1	14q12	AD	MYH7 (myosin H chain)	192600
CMH2	1q32	AD	TNNT2 (Troponin T)	115195
CMH3	15q22.1	AD	TPM1 (α-tropomyosin)	115196
CMH4	11p11.2	AD	MYBPC3	115197
CMH5	?	AD	?	115198
CMH6	7q31-qter	AD	?	600858
CMH7	19q13.4	AD	TNNI3 (Troponin I)	191044
CMH8	3p	AD	MYL3 (myosin L chain)	160790
CMH9	2q24.3	AD	TTN (Titin)	188840
	14q12	AD	MYH6 (myosin H chain)	160710
	20q13.3	AD	MYLK2	606566
	15q14	AD	ACTC (Actin)	102540
	12q23-q24.3	AD	MYL2 (myosin L chain)	160781
CMH/WPW	7q36	AD	PRKAG2	600858
	9q34	AD	GSN (Gelsolin)	137350
	Xq22	XR	GLA (α-Galactosidase)	301500
	MtDNA	mt	TRNA-Gly	590035
	MtDNA	mt	TRNA-Lys	590060

Subsequent detection of causative mutations in MYH7 opened the way to systematic investigations on other candidate genes, selected on the basis of participation of corresponding proteins to the contractile machinery of myocardial cell.

Research, which involved several groups, was extremely successful. Presently CMH may be considered on the cutting edge of investigation in molecular genetics applied to Cardiology. Not only several genes and many causative mutations were identified, but molecular genetics investigation is proceeding further.

Expression profiling data started to be produced. In the heart of patients affected with CMH, a series of genes appeared upregulated; among these, genes encoding cytoskeletal proteins, redox system components and ion channels were identified (Lim, 2001).

Identification of causative mutation is becoming part of diagnostic procedure. Moreover, clinical evaluation and follow-up of carriers of given mutations started to produce unbiased data on inter- and intra-familial variability of clinical presentation, severity and disease progression, which are very important for assessing individual risk in probands.

The most frequent type of CMH is CMH1 (35-50% of the total), followed by CMH2 (15-20%) and by CMH4 (15-20%). Each of the other forms account for less than 5% of the total.

Over 100 mutations have been identified so far. The majority of them are point mutations, although deletions, insertions and splice mutations are often reported in MYBPC3.

Most CMH mutations arise independently, thus almost every family has a "private" mutation. A regularly updated collection of data on mutations associated with CMH phenotypes is available at the website http://www.angis.org.au/Databases/Heart/heartbreak.html .

In several cases, genotype-phenotype studies provided interesting results about "benignity" or "malignity" of some forms or of some peculiar mutations.

For instance, it was possible to establish that in forms due to mutation of β-myosin heavy chain, the degree of hypertrophy positively correlates with risk of sudden death. On the contrary, in mutations of Troponin T, there is high risk of sudden death, even in cases of mild or absent hypertrophy. Mutations in Myosin-binding protein C are usually associated with rather benign clinical course: risk of sudden death is low and progressive hypertrophy develops late.

Some mutations may appear as benign in heterozygotes, but they cause a very severe phenotype in the homozygote, as shown by Ser179Phe mutation in cardiac Troponin T (Ho, 2000).

Intrafamilial variability may be ascribed to environmental factors (physical exercise due to demanding jobs or to sport activity), to cardiovascular alterations (e.g. hypertension), or to differences in individual genetic background.

In some families a peculiar type of CMH (OMIM 600858) was described, associated with Wolff-Parkinson White syndrome (WPW, OMIM 194200). Causative mutations were detected in PRKAG2 gene, encoding gamma-2 subunit of AMP-activated protein kinase. On the other hand, WPW was observed in individuals with Gly203Ser mutation in gene encoding cardiac troponin I and in one person carrying a 2-nt deletion at codon 945 in MYBPC3 gene, encoding Myosin-binding protein C3.

Hypertrophic cardiomyopathy was found in cases affected with Leigh syndrome (LS, OMIM 256000). Left-sided obstructive cardiomyopathy is reported in Leopard syndrome (OMIM 151100).

Cardiomyopathy with left ventricular hypertrophy and aortic root dilatation was described in Familial amyloidosis, Finnish type, due to mutation in GSN gene, encoding Gelsolin (OMIM 137350) and in Acyl-CoA dehydrogenase, very long chain, deficiency (VLCAD, autosomal recessive, OMIM 201475).

CMH due to mutation of mitochondrial transfer RNA for Lysine (OMIM 590060) was described, associated with deafness, in MERRF syndrome (Myoclonic Epilepsy with Ragged Red Fibers). Non-obstructive CMH was reported in a family carrying a mutation of mitochondrial tRNA for Glycine. CMH may be caused also by mutations in genes coding for other mitochondrial tRNAs.

Dilated cardiomyopathy (CMD= CardioMyopathy, Dilated) is possibly the most frequent cause of cardiac heart failure, with a prevalence of 4-5/10,000.

The main feature of CMD is the enlargement of ventricular chambers, associated to reduced contractility. In general, disease is manifested in the adult, between 18 and 50 years of age.

The incidence of the disease is underestimated, since asymptomatic cases escape detection and benign forms are often misdiagnosed. Over 40% of patients affected with CMD show a positive familar history for the disease. Phenocopies may be encountered.

Familial CMDs are genetically heterogeneous: some forms are transmitted as autosomal dominant traits, others as autosomal recessives. X-linked recessive inheritance and mitochondrial inheritance were described as well (Tab.4.2).

Current OMIM classification reports 13 different genetic types of CMD. CMD1B, CMD1D, CMD1G and CMD1K are reported as "pure" forms, while CMD1A, CMD1E, CMD1F , CMD1H and CMD1I are characterized by presence of conduction defects. CMDF, CMDI and CMDL are associated with skeletal myopathies.

The peculiarity of this association with skeletal muscle disorders is confirmed by the observation that dilative cardiomyopathy occurs as a part of the clinical phenotype in Duchenne and Becker X-linked muscular dystrophies. Cases of severe dilative cardiomyopathy were occasionally reported in female carriers of this disease (Melacini, 1998).

It is interesting to notice that some Dystrophin mutations can cause dilative cardiomyopathy with minimal or none skeletal muscle involvement (Towbin, 1993; Muntoni, 1993; Milasin, 1996; Ortiz-Lopez, 1997).

Several genes whose mutations lead to dilative cardiomyopathy code for proteins participating in complex systems of structural relationships linking extracellular matrix and intercellular junctions to sarcomere, inner cytoskeleton and nuclear envelope (δ-sarcoglycan, dystrophin, titin, desmoplakin, actin, myosin, troponin, tropomyosin, desmin, lamin).

Table 4.2 : Genetic heterogeneity of CMDs. (I: mode of inheritance; AD: autosomal dominant; AR: autosomal recessive; XL: X-linked; mt: carried by mitochondrial DNA)

Type	Locus	I	Gene	OMIM
CMD1A	1q21.2	AD	Lamin A/C	115200
CMD1G	2q31	AD	TTN (Titin)	604145
CMD11	2q35	AD	DES (Desmin)	604765
CMD1L	5q33-q34	AR	SGCD (δ-sarcoglycan)	606685
CMD3A	Xq28	XR	G4.5 (?)	300069
	14q12	AD	MYH7 (myosin H chain)	160760
	14q11.2-q12	AD	TNNT2 (Troponin)	191045
	15q14	AD	ACTC (Actin)	102540
	15q22.1	AD	TPM1αTropomyosin	191010
	Xq28	XR	G4.5	302060
	6p24	AR	DSP (Desmoplakin)	605676
	Xp21	XR	DYS (Dystrophin)	300376
	9q13	AR	FRDA (Frataxin)	229300
	18cen-q12.3	AD	TTR (Transthyretin)	176300
	Xp21.1	XR	XK (McLeod)	314850
	17q25.2-q25.3	AR	GAA (acid maltase)	232300
	MtDNA	mt	KSS (Kearns-Sayre)	530000
	MtDNA	mt	tRNA-His	590040
	MtDNA	mt	tRNA-Ileu	590045
	MtDNA	mt	tRNA-Leu	590050
	MtDNA	mt	tRNA-Lys	590060

It has been suggested that alteration in any of these proteins would cause reduction in force generated by contractile machinery, since cytoskeleton imposes a resistive intracellular load on sarcomere.

mtDNA mutations, causing impairment of energy production, would also reduce the force generated by the sarcomere, both in cardiac and skeletal muscle. Association of dilative cardiomyopathy with skeletal muscle symptoms is often observed in mitochondrial disorders.

Noticeably, mutation in sarcomeric protein-encoding genes actin, βMHC, α-Tropomyosin, and cardiac Troponin T may either cause CMD or hypertrophic cardiomyopathy. Individuals affected with CMD1I may show concentric and obstructive ventricular hypertrophy.

Table 4.3: CMDs in which involved genes are still unknown. (I: mode of inheritance; AD: autosomal dominant; AR: autosomal recessive)

Type	Locus	I	Features	OMIM
CMD1B	9q13-q22	AD	Pure CMD	600884
CMD1C	10q21-q23	AD	Mitral prolapse/LVD	601493
CMD1D	1q32	AD	Pure CMD/ LVD	601494
CMD1E	3p25-p22	AD	CDCD2/stroke	601154
CMD1F	6q23	AD	CDCD3/LGMD	602067
CMD1H	2q14-q22	AD	CDCD/Vtachycardia	604288
CMD1J	6q23-q24	AD	Hearing loss	605362
CMD1K	6q12-q16	AD	Pure CMD/LVD	605582
	1p1-1q1	AD	Atrial CM with heart block	108770
	?	AR	Pure CMD (?)	212110
	?	AR	Microcephaly-Cardiomyopathy	251220
	?	AR	Congestive CM/hypogonadism	212112

Tab. 4.3 reports a series of dilative cardiomyopathies for which the involved gene is still unknown. In some of them, dilated cardiomyopathy is

the main clinical feature, while in others cardiac affection is part of the clinical phenotype. In Barth's syndrome (OMIM 302060), dilated cardiomyopathy is associated with endocardial fibroelastosis, which, on the other hand, was reported as single entity, inherited as X-linked recessive trait (OMIM 305300). It is still unclear if this form could be included within the spectrum of Barth's phenotype.

Restrictive cardiomyopathy (OMIM 115210) is a rare condition, characterized by diastolic dysfunction and atrial enlargement without ventricular dilatation. It occurs rarely as a " pure" familial form, inherited as autosomal dominant trait. Thus far, only 4 families were reported in the literature, in which genetic and clinical investigations were adequate (Fitzpatrick, 1990; Katritsis, 1991; Feld, 1992; Ishiwata, 1993). In one of such families variable hypertrophic and restrictive features were observed.

On the other hand, non-hypertrophic restrictive cardiomyopathy was described in association with Noonan's syndrome (OMIM 163950), by Cooke et al.(1994).

Evidence in favour of a familial form of idiopathic restrictive cardiomyopathy was reviewed by Kushawa (1997).

Cases of restrictive cardiomyopathy were seldom observed in Cardioskeletal Desmin-related myopathy (OMIM 601419), inherited as autosomal dominant, in Pseudoxantoma elasticum (OMIM 264800, autosomal recessive), in Fabry's disease (OMIM 301500, α-Galactosidase deficiency, X-linked recessive), and in Aminoglycoside-induced deafness, due to mutation (A1555G) of 12S mitochondrial rRNA (OMIM 561000).

Arrhythmogenic Right Ventricular Cardiomyopathy (ARVC, formerly ARVD: Arrhythmogenic Right Ventricular Dysplasia, OMIM 107970) is a recently established group of diseases (McKenna, 1994). characterized by progressive degeneration of the right ventricular myocardium, associated with severe arrhythmias and increased risk of sudden cardiac death, especially in teenagers and in young adults.

Reviews on this genetic disorder were produced by Thiene (1997), Fontaine (1999), and Danieli (2002).

ARVCs are still often unrecognized and misdiagnosed. Most cases are detected at the autopsy, because of gross findings (thinning of the right ventricular free wall, massive fibro-fatty substitution of the myocardial tissue). However, since necropsy is seldom performed in cases of sudden cardiac death over 35 years of age, autopsy cases may possibly represent the tip of an iceberg. Moreover, several affected individuals may escape detection even in families with a previous positive history for the disease, since ARVC is inherited as autosomal dominant trait with reduced penetrance.

Prevalence of ARVC is presently estimated between 5/1,000 and 6/10,000.

Linkage analysis succeeded in identifying several different ARVC loci independently involved in determination of the disease (Tab. 4.4). Probably, genetic heterogeneity in ARVCs is even larger, since in several families linkage with any of the known loci was excluded.

Involved genes were identified so far only in two ARVC forms. In Naxos disease, an autosomal recessive disorder where arrhythmogenic right ventricular cardiomyopathy associates with palmoplantar keratoderma and woolly hairs, a homozygous frame-shift mutation (due to 2-nt deletion) was detected in the Plakoglobin gene (McKoy, 2000). Plakoglobin is a key component of desmosomes and adherens junctions, involved in tight adhesion of many cell types, cardiomyocytes included.

Causative mutations of ARVC2 were detected in the RYR2 gene (encoding cardiac ryanodine receptor). ARVC2 is characterized by polymorphic effort-induced ventricular tachyarrhythmias, high risk of sudden death in asymptomatic individuals and by variable degree of myocardial degeneration (Tiso el al., 2001).

Table 4.4 : Genetic heterogeneity of ARVCs (I: mode of inheritance; AD: autosomal dominant; AR: autosomal recessive). Types still retain the old acronym "ARVD"

Type	Locus	I	Gene	OMIM
ARVD1	14q23-q24	AD	?	107970
ARVD2	1q42-q43	AD	RYR2 (Ryanodine receptor)	600996
ARVD3	14q12-q22	AD	?	602086
ARVD4	2q32	AD	?	602087
ARVD5	3p23	AD	?	604400
ARVD6	10p12	AD	?	604401
ARVD7	10q22	AD	?	unavailable
Naxos	17	AR	JUP (Plakoglobin)	188840

Interestingly, mutations in the same gene were reported in catecholaminergic polymorphic ventricular tachycardia (alias VTA: Ventricular Tachycardia, Arrhythmogenic) (Priori, 2001). It is still unclear if differences in clinical phenotypes formerly defined respectively as ARVC2 and VTA might be due to individual phenotypic variability or to functional differences in specific mutations of the same gene.

4.2 Genetic heterogeneity of cardiomyopathies and the "final common pathway" hypothesis

A striking feature of inherited cardiomyopathies is their broad genetic heterogeneity, concomitant with ample phenotype variability, even within diseases due to mutations of the same gene.

Original classification of cardiomyopathies was mainly based on gross phenotype description. Basically, hypertrophic forms were separated from dilated and from restrictive forms, respectively. The discovery of genes involved in these disease produced the unpleasant feeling that present classification is shaking, since mutations in the same gene may determine different diseases (e.g. hypertrophic or dilated cardiomyopathy), as well as mutations in different genes may produce the "same" disease.

Mendelian genetics, developed when the material nature of genes and mutations was totally unknown, produced an oversimplified view of genetic disease: one mutation in one gene produces one phenotype. Even A. Garrod, the imaginative founder of biochemical genetics, was unable to figure the complexity of biochemical relationships leading to clinical phenotype.

In early times, medical genetics was dealing almost exclusively with diseases showing full penetrance and little inter-individual variability in the clinical phenotype. For this reason, the false impression of simple genotype-phenotype relationships was fixed.

On the contrary, now we are fully aware that clinical phenotype is the ultimate result of one (or more) defect(s) involving important or fundamental component(s) of a very complex biochemical network underlying cellular, tissue and organ function. Therefore, we understand why a defect in any relevant component of the network underlying a specific function could be pathogenic.

Recently, this idea has been shaped into the "final common pathway" hypothesis (Towbin, 2001), particularly useful for approaching the complexity of cardiomyopathies.

Let's start from the most simple example. Mutations in some genes (several tRNAs and one rRNA) carried by mitochondrial DNA produce cardiomyopathy (hypertrophic or dilated). It is intuitive that a defect in the machinery generating ATP would be harmful to cardiomyocyte, which needs a continuous supply of energy, even when the body is at rest. Therefore any mutation in mtDNA is expected to be pathogenic to the heart. The relatively low number of mutations described so far may be due to a bias in investigations (not all laboratories are experienced in mtDNA research) or, more probably, to lethality of some mutations in early stages of development.

Anyway, the identification of mtDNA mutations associated with cardiomyopathies demonstrated that a normal cardiac phenotype needs of the functional integrity of the energy production module.

The same concept applies to other functional modules.

Table 4.5: Major proteins involved in myocardiocyte contractile machinery

Proteins	Function
Z-disk	
Actin	Contraction
β-actinin	Actin-capping
α-actinin	Actinin cross-linking
CAPZ	Actin-capping
α-Crystallin	Desmin binding
M-line	
Myosin	Contraction
M protein	Myosin binding
C protein	Myosin binding
Creatine kinase	Energy transduction
Titin	Actin/myosin setting

Contractile machinery is the core of myocardiocyte function. What we call "contraction" is the effect of molecular mechanics, based on sliding of contractile proteins (Tab. 4.5). A defect in one component of such machinery is expected to reduce efficiency of contraction.

On the other hand, cytoskeleton (another functional module with several different components) is deeply inter-related and inter-connected with the contraction molecular machinery. Therefore, it may be expected that also a defective cytoskeletal protein would result in a decreased contractile performance.

Table 4.6: Major proteins involved in connections of myocardiocytes

Protein	Function
α-actinin	Linking vinculin/actin
β-dystroglycan	Linking dystrophin to basal membrane
A-CAM	Linking adjacent cells across extracellular space
Connexins	Constituent intercellular channels (connexons)
Desmoglein	Constituent of desmosomes
Desmoplakin	Constituent of desmosomes
Dystrophin	Linking actin/β-dystroglycan
Integrin	Transmembrane linking collagen/talin
Plakoglobin	Constituent of desmosomes
Plakoglobulin	Binding A-CAM/Vinculin
Talin	Linking integrin/vinculin
Vinculin	Linking talin/α-actinin
Vinculin	Linking α-catenin/α-actinin

Connection between cardiomyocytes and with extracellular matrix, corresponds to another functional module, involving structures due to interaction of several different proteins (Tab. 4.6) which, in turn, are connected to cytoskeleton.

In cardiomyocytes, intercalated disks show three different types of junctional specialized structures: *Macula adherens* (desmosomes), *Fascia adherens* and "tight junctions". Several proteins co-operate in building such structures. Also costamere adherens junctions involve interactions of a series of proteins. Again, a defect in any of these proteins involved in intercellular connection or in connection to extracellular matrix is expected to be harmful to myocardial cell physiological performance.

The so-called " ionic channels" correspond to a functional module regulating ionic exchange across membranes. This module is of primary importance for myocardiocyte physiology, since it provides the ground for excitation-contraction coupling and intracellular and inter-cellular signalling.

Coming back to cardiomyopathies, dilated forms seem to derive mostly from defective sarcomere anchorage to cytoskeleton, while hypetrophic cardiomyopathies are mostly due to defective contraction machinery and arrhythmogenic right ventricular cardiomyopathies possibly result from defects in intercellular connections (Fig. 4.1).

However, it is too early for drawing firm conclusions, since we do not know yet all proteins involved in such processes. Some "missing links" might clarify why mutations in some genes show alternative phenotypes. Moreover, present knowledge about disease phenotypes is strongly biased: usually, once a mutation is detected, which could reasonably explain the origin of the considered disease, mutations in additional genes are not searched for. On the contrary, possible concomitant presence of a mutation with relatively small pathogenic effect, in a different gene, might reasonably explain the occurrence of peculiar and unusual disease phenotypes.

We should remember that, even in physiological conditions, heart undergoes remodelling, as a consequence of mechanical overload. Nature and implications of cardiac and vascular remodelling were clearly treated by Swyngedauw (1998) in a very informative book on molecular cardiology.

In cardiomyopathies, remodelling is adversely affected by genetically altered performance of cardiomyocytes, fibrosis and cell deaths. Effect of defective genes on remodelling has been not adequately investigated in detail so far.

At present, "final common pathway" hypothesis is the frame in which knowledge on gene defects is gradually reconstituting the overall picture of pathogenesis in cardiomyopathies. Moreover, this working hypothesis provides a rationale for a shortcut in the long processs of identification of genes involved in diseases. Some genes may be suspected by function ("functional cloning"), and thus submitted to mutation screening, bypassing linkage analysis.

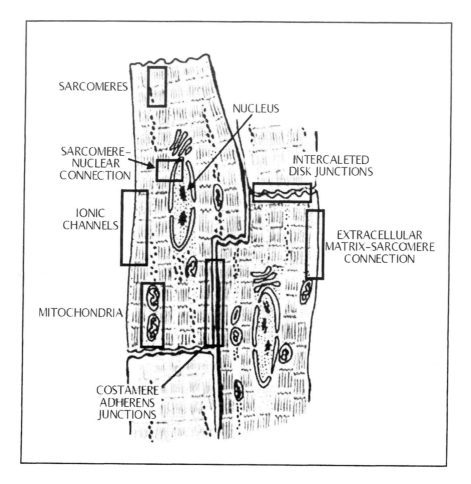

Figure 4.1 : Main cardiomyocyte functional modules, targeted by mutations leading to cardiomyopathy. (from Brobeck, modified)

4.3 Arrhythmic disorders

Arrhythmias are commonly observed in congenital heart defects and in cardiomyopathies (Tab. 4.7).

Table 4.7 : Cardiac arrhythmias associated with structural heart diseases (AF: atrial fibrillation; AVB: atrio-ventricular block; BBB: bundle-branch block; VT: ventricular tachycardia; AD: autosomal dominant; AR: autosomal recessive; XL: X-linked; mt: carried by mitochondrial DNA) (From Roberts, 2000, modified)

Type	Disease	Rhythm	Inheritance
SV	Familiar amyloidosls	AF	AD
V	CMHs	AF/VT	AD,mt
	CMH/WPW	AF/VT	AD
	Naxos disease	VT	AR
	ARVDs	VT	AD
	CMD	VT	AD,AR,XL, mt
	Mitral valve prolapse	AF	AD
CD	Restrictive CM	AVB	AD
	Familial amyloidosis	AVB	AD
	Holt-Oram syndrome	AVB/AT	AD
	Atrial septal defect	AVB, BBB	AD

Arrhythmic disorders associated to different neuromuscular diseases were described (Tab. 4.8). In the past, this kind of association was reported occasionally. More recently, specific studies were conducted, in order to fully evaluate heart involvement in neuromuscular disorders (Melacini, 1996,1999), since in patients affected with severe neuromuscular disorders not only survival, but also quality of life might greatly benefit from a proper cardiac treatment.

Table 4.8 : Cardiac arrhythmias associated with neuromuscular disorders (AF: atrial fibrillation ; AT: atrial tachycardia ; AVB: atrio-ventricular block ; VT : ventricular tachycardia; AD: autosomal dominant; AR: autosomal recessive; XL: X-linked; mt: carried by mitochondrial DNA) (From Roberts, 2000, modified)

Disease	Rhythm	Inheritance
Barth syndrome	AT/VT	XL
Becker	AVB	XL
Duchenne	AT/AVB	XL
Emery-Dreyfuss	AF	XL
Friedreich ataxia	Variable	AR
FSH	AF	AD
Kearn-Sayre	AVB	mt
Kugelberg-welander	AF/AVB	AR
LGDs	AVB	AR
McArdle	AVB	AR,AD
Myotonic dystrophy	AVB/VT	AD

Although arrhythmias are often part of different disease phenotypes, there are genetically inherited arrhythmias showing no evidence of structural heart disease, nor concomitant presence of an additional genetic disorder. They are usually referred as "primary cardiac arrhythmias" or "pure" inherited cardiac arrhythymias. They may show supraventricular or ventricular origin or may be due to conduction defects. Tab. 4.9 provides a general summarized information

At the end of previous section, we have seen that, according to the "final common pathway" hypothesis, we should expect that genetically inherited alterations of heartbeat could occur as a consequence of defective regulation of ionic exchange across membranes. This is actually the case.

Table 4.9: Cardiac arrhythmias with no structural heart disease (AF: atrial fibrillation; AVB: Atrio-ventricular block; AVRT: atrio-ventricular re-entrant tachycardia; CD: Conduction defect; RBBB: right-bundle-branch block; SV: supra-ventricular; TdP: "torsade de pointes"; V: ventricular; VF: ventricular fibrillation; VT: ventricular tachycardia; AD: autosomal dominant; AR: autosomal recessive) (From Roberts, 2000, modified)

Type	Disease	Rhythm	Inheritance
SV	Atrial fibrillation	AF	AD
	Atrial stand-still	SND/AF	AD
	WPW	AVRT	AD
	Familial PJRT	AVRT	AD
V	LQT syndrome (RW)	TdP	AD
	LQT syndrome (JLN)	TdP	AR
	Familial VT	VT	AD
	Bi-directional VT	VT	AD
	Brugada syndrome	VT/VF	AD
CD	Atrio-ventricular block	AVB	AD
	Familial BBB	RBBB	?

The first locus for autosomal dominant Long-QT syndrome was discovered in 1991. Since then, additional genes involved in dominantly inherited L-QT syndromes have been identified through the effects of their mutations (Tab. 4.10). Surprisingly, Jervell and Lange-Nielsen syndrome, inherited as autosomal recessive and associated with deafness, was found to be due to homozygosity for mutations in genes involved in L-QT1 and L-QT5. Estimated prevalence of LQT syndrome is about 1/10,000. The disease may cause sudden cardiac death. LQT3 was recently linked to sudden infant death syndrome (Schwartz, 2000) .

Table 4.10 : Genetic heterogeneity of Long-QT syndrome. (I: mode of inheritance; AD: autosomal dominant; AR: autosomal recessive)

Type	Locus	I	Gene	OMIM
LQT1	11p15.5	AD	KCNQ1	192500
LQT2	7q35-q36	AD	KCNH2	152427
LQT3	3p21	AD	SCN5A	603830
LQT4	4q25-q27	AD	?	600919
LQT5	21q22.1-q22.2	AD	KCNE1 (MINK)	176261
LQT6	21q22.1-q22.2	AD	KCNE2 (MIRP1)	603796
JLNS1	11p15.5/21q21.2-q22.2	AR	KCNQ1/KCNE1	220400

Comprehensive reviews on genetic and molecular basis of Long-QT syndromes were provided by Priori (1999) and Dumaine (2002).

All L-QT syndromes known so far are due to defects in sodium channel (SNC5A) or in potassium channels. Mutations in SNC5a produce an increased Na^+ flux, whereas mutations in K^+ channels determine loss of function.

The result of mutations is a perturbation of inward/outward current balance during the plateau of the action potential. Fig. 4.2 shows the structure of the involved channels and the electrocardiographic consequences of their defects.

In all forms of L-QT syndromes, prolongation of repolarization time may produce polymorphic ventricular tachycardia in the form "torsade de pointes" and, eventually, sudden death.

A comprehensive review on cardiac "channelopathies" was given by Marban (2002). Interestingly, mutations of SCN5A gene may cause Brugada syndrome (autosomal dominant, OMIM 601144), characterized by right bundle branch block and ST segment elevation, idiopathic fibrillation and high risk of cardiac arrest and sudden death.

High prevalence of Brugada syndrome is reported in South East Asia and Japan. A review on clinical features of this disease was produced by Alings (1999) , on a series of 163 cases reported in the literature.

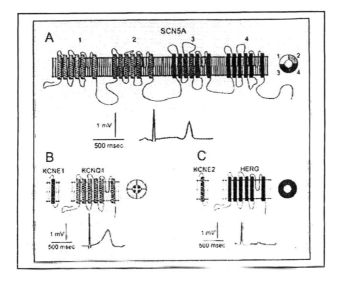

Figure 4.2 : Structure of ion channels involved in L-QT syndromes and electrocardiograms corresponding to specific genetic defects (A= LQT3; B=LQT1; C=LQT2). (from Dumaine, modified)

As shown in Fig. 4.3., ionic balance controlled by sodium and potassium channels is inter-related with maintainance of intracellular calcium concentration.

Intracellular calcium concentration is under different and stringent controls (Mackrill, 1999).

Excitation promotes a modest Cu^{++} influx across cardiomyocyte plasma membrane, through dihydropyridine receptor. This Ca^{++} influx activates ryanodyne receptors, thus determinig the immediate release of Ca^{++} from calcium stores of sarcoplasmic reticulum and consequent contraction of sarcomere. After contraction, SERCA removes Ca^{++} from sarcomere and cytoplasm, concentrating it within sarcoplasmic reticulum stores, with the help of specific Ca++binding proteins.

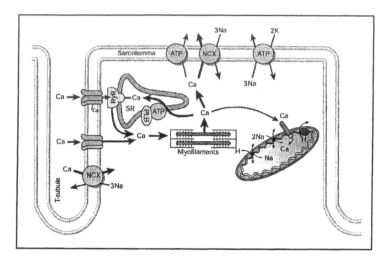

Figure 4.3 : Calcium transport in ventricular cardiomyocytes (ATP: ATPase; PLB: Phospholamban; RyR: Ryanodine receptor; NCX: Sodium channel; SR: Sarcoplasmic reticulum). (From Bers, modified)

Excessive intracellular calcium concentration would activate proteases, induce leaking of Cytochrome C from mitochondria and trigger apoptosis. Therefore, a defect in proteins involved in control of intracellular calcium concentration may produce several harmful effects to cardiomyocytes, beside alteration of excitation-contraction coupling. In an excellent overview on genetic basis of cardiomyopathies (Seidman, 2001), the role of calcium in development of cardiac hypertrophy and dilation was considered.

Recently, mutations in RYR2 gene, encoding human cardiac ryanodine receptor protein, were detected in cases of ARVD2 (arrhythmogenic right ventricular cardiomyopathy, type 2, see this Chapter, section 4.4) and in cases of stress-induced ventricular tachycardia (VTA, autosomal dominant, OMIM

604772), providing clear evidence that a defect in Ryanodine Calcium channel may produce arrhythmic disease.

A database of gene mutations in arrhythmic disorders is available (http://PC4.FSM.it:81/cardmoc/homepage.htm).

Few additional arrhythmic disorders are reported in OMIM, still waiting for identification of the involved genes (Tab. 4.11).

Table 4.11: Inherited arrhythmic disorders still waiting for identification of the involved gene(s).

Disease	Locus	OMIM
Atrial fibrillation with bradyarrhythmia	?	163800
Atrial tachyarrhythmia with short PR interval	?	108950
Cardiac conduction defect with sudden death	?	115080
Progressive familial heart block, Type I	3p21	113900
Progressive familial heart block, Type I,I	19q13.2-q13.3	604559
Progressive familial heart block, Type II	?	140400
Ventricular fibrillation, Paroxysmal familia	3p21	603829

On the other hand, many channels are known to be active in the heart (see Appendix III). Some of them might be possibly involved in arrhythmic inherited disorders still waiting for the discovery of causative gene mutations.

Research in this field is very active. It is possible that in the next five years not only genes involved in arrhythmogenic disorders, but almost all genes involved in cardiac monogenic diseases could be identified.

This novel situation will probably open new avenues to treatment. In fact, knowledge of molecular defects underlying given diseases will prompt testing of suitable drugs in vitro and in animal models.

Moreover, some already available drugs might possibly reveal therapeutical efficacy on selected diseases or disease variants. Finally, therapeutic trials, conducted on cohorts of patients sharing the same genetic defect, are expected to produce sharp results, thus reducing the time needed for clinical experimentation.

4.4 Genetic basis of congenital heart defects in humans

Congenital heart diseases in humans frequently involve abnormalities at cardiac subcompartment boundaries, malformations of cardiac outlet connections, or abnormal chamber remodelling.

Most common congenital human heart diseases are: atrial septal defects, ventricular septal defects, persistency of the atrioventricular canal, persistency of the truncus arteriosus, transposition of great vessels, dextrocardia and Tetralogy of Fallot.

Until recently, it was widely accepted that about 2% of congenital heart diseases were due to teratogens, 8% to single-gene defects and 90% of multifactorial origin, however, mutations determining development of phenotypes mimicking human congenital heart diseases were characterized so far in different organisms, from fruitfly to African clawed toad , zebrafish and mouse. Moreover, an increasing number of genes whose mutations cause heart diseases is being identified in humans.

Mutations in cardiac-specific homeo-box gene CSX (OMIM 600584) were detected in families with atrial septal defect (ASD, OMIM 108800, prevalence 1:10,000), with atrial septal defect and atrioventicular conduction defects (OMIM 108900; CSX, Thr178Met; Gln170ter; Gln198ter), with tetralogy of Fallot (OMIM 187500; CSX Arg25Cys; Glu21Gln; Ala219Val) or with idiopathic second-degree atrio-ventricular block (CSX,IVS1DSG-T,+1). Phenotypic effects of CSX mutations are inherited as autosomal dominant traits with reduced penetrance and noticeable phenotypic variability.

Mutations in TBX5, a T-box gene mapped to 12q24.1, were shown to cause Holt-Oram syndrome (OMIM 142900), a rare autosomal dominant disorder characterized by thumb anomalies and atrial septal defect. In some cases ventricular septal defect may be present. T-box gene codes for a transcription factor. Interestingly, some mutations (e.g. Gly80Arg) cause significant cardiac malformations but only minor limb abnormalities, whereas others (e.g. Arg237Gln and Arg237Trp) produce gross upper limb malformations, but less significant cardiac anomalies.

Studies in large families showing atrial septal defects succeeded in discovering the involvement of gene NKX2.5, encoding a different transcription factor, expressed both in the atrial septum and in the conduction tissue.

Left ventricular noncompaction (LVNC, OMIM 606617) is characterized by deep trabeculations in the left ventricular endocardium, associated with left ventricular hypertrophy, dilation or hypertrophy and dilatation. Heart appears thick, with a dilated chamber, i.e. hypertrophic and dilated. Main feature is systolic dysfunction. In some cases right ventricle may be affected as well. The defect was thought to be due to arrest in myocardial morphogenesis.

Familial forms of LVNC may be found associated with septal defects, hypoplastic left ventricle or with pulmonary stenosis. Some cases are due to mutations in G4.5 gene (X-linked, involved in Barth's syndrome , OMIM 302060).

A case of Left ventricular noncompaction with congenital heart defects, due to mutation in α-dystrobrevin, participating in the dystrophin-associated sarcolemmal protein complex, has been reported (OMIM 601239). Involvement of dystrobrevin would suggest an alteration of connection between extracellular matrix and inner cytoskeleton. On the other hand, since dystrobrevin n-terminal domain is associated with sarcoglycan-sarcospan complex, supposedly linked to nitric oxide synthase, the possibility of defective intracellular signulling produced by α-dystrobrevin mutations cannot be excluded. A Left ventricular noncompaction, isolated form (OMIM 604169), inherited as autosomal dominant trait, was also described.

Situs inversus viscerum (OMIM 270100) is a rare congenital affection characterized by reversed anatomical position of asymmetric visceral organs, heart included. Most cases are sporadic. Autosomal dominant, autosomal recessive and X-linked inheritance were reported, suggesting strong genetic heterogeneity. One disease locus was mapped to 9p13-p21.

Gross cardiovascular anomalies are present also in Asplenia and Polysplenia (OMIM 208530, inherited as autosomal recessive trait).

DiGeorge syndrome (OMIM 188400) and Velocardiofacial syndrome (VCFS, OMIM 192430) are rare autosomal dominant disorders asssociated with interstitial deletions of the long arm of chromosome 22, in the region 22q11. Clinical phenotype is variable: cardiac features include tetralogy of Fallot, interruption of the aortic arc, persistency of truncus arteriosus and ventricular septal defect.

Gene(s) involved in Di George and velocardiofacial syndromes still remains unidentified. Variability in clinical phenotypes is ascribed to variable extension of the deleted segment, whic implies variation in the number of genes included in the deletion.

Williams syndrome (mapped to 7q11.2, OMIM 194050) phenotype is characterized by peculiar facies, neonatal hypercalciemia and mental retardation, associated with heart defects including supravalvular aortic stenosis, pulmonary valve stenosis and, in some cases, coronary obstructive lesions. Defects seem to be caused by mutations in elastin gene, inherited as autosomal dominant traits.

Alagille syndrome (autosomal dominant, mapped to 20p12, OMIM 118450) is characterized by neonatal jaundice (deficiency of intrahepatic bile ducts), associated with peripheral pulmonary artery stenosis, atrial and/or ventricular septal defect, aortic coarctation. This disorder is caused by mutations in the Jagged1 gene, encoding the ligand of Notch receptor, involved in signalling pathway in early development.

Finally, Char syndrome (autosomal dominant, mapped to6p12, OMIM 169100), showing craniofacial abnormalities and patent ductus arteriosus, is due to mutations in gene TFAP2B, encoding a transcription factor and expressed in the neural crest.

4.5 Transgenic animals and the genetic dissection of developmental phenotypes

The most profitable approach used so far for understanding genetic determination of complex phenotype is "genetic dissection". Actually, analysis of phenotypic effect of mutations in single genes, helps in deciphering the contribution of each gene to normal phenotype. For instance, if mutation in a specific gene produces a noticeable alteration at a given stage and in a given tissue or organ, this would tell us that protein coded by such a gene is needed, at that stage and in that tissue, for normal development.

Most of present knowledge about the development of heart is due to studies conducted on mice. In the past, analysis was limited to naturally occurring mutants, but in recent years molecular genetics methods, coupled with techniques of cell manipulation and gene transfer, enabled scientists to produce artificial mutants in mice, thus tremendously expanding the power of this approach.

A "transgenic" is an animal whose cells carry an artificially introduced DNA segment. In order to create it, it is necessary to insert the gene selected to be transferred (the "transgene") into a fertilized oocyte or in embryonic stem cells (ES cells). In such a way, all or most somatic and germinal cells of the resulting organism will carry the transgene. If gene transfer was successful and transgene was stably integrated in the genome, the animal could show a novel phenotype or, more simply, it may express a novel protein, coded by the transgene.

In mice, it is possible to mutagenize a selected gene in vitro and transfer mutant copies to cultured ES cells isolated from blastocyst of a given non-mutant strain, or to artificially substitute normal copies of a given gene with mutant ones, as described later.

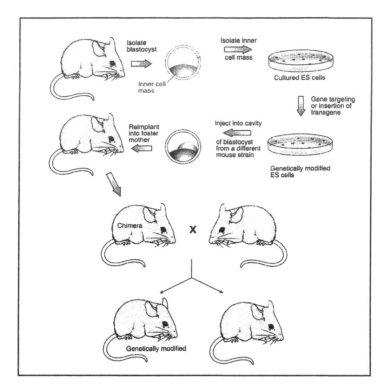

Figure 4.4: Creation of a transgenic mouse, by ES cells manipulation and subsequent backcross (see text for explanation). (From Strachan & Read, modified)

As shown in Fig.4.4, manipulated ES cells, originally obtained from a given mouse strain, are injected into the cavity of a blastocyst from a different mouse strain. Blastocyst is then implanted into a foster mother of a known strain, where development takes place. The resulting newborn mouse will be a "chimera" , i.e. a mixture of cells derived from two lineages: those from original blastocyst cells, and those derived from manipulated ES cells. Presence of lineages of cells derived from those in which gene transfer was successful and followed by stable integration into the host genome may be assessed by simple PCR tests, performed on DNA samples from tiny tissue specimens (e.g. tail tips).

Once recognized, chimeric individuals are then backcrossed. Occasionally, chimera's germinal cells may derive from ES manipulated cells. In these cases crossing will produce mice heterozygous for the artificially transferred mutation. Subsequent inbreeding of such heterozygotes will produce mice homozygotes for the selected mutation.

Genomic integration of transgenes occurs at random, but techniques (site-specific recombination systems) are available for inserting a transgene in a specific genomic sequence (Fig. 4.5).

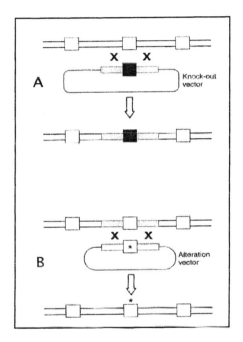

Figure 4.5: Gene targeting. Gene replacement (A) or substitution of normal allele by a mutant copy (B) may be achieved by homologous recombination between a specific genomic region and a DNA segment carried by a vector. X indicate the flanking sites where recombination occurs. (From Strachan & Read, modified)

Gene targeting may be used to produce insertional mutations in pre-selected genes, or to replace genes with their mutant copies.

By this procedure it is possible to "knock-out" a specific gene and even to construct "double knock-out" mice, i.e. homozygotes for two different gene defects, or to produce individuals homozygotes or heterozygotes for a given mutation.

Therefore, by transgenesis and gene targeting it is possible to create animal models of selected human diseases. While modelling a loss-of-function is achieved by gene knock-out, gain-of-function is usually modelled by inserting a mutant copy of the gene involved in the disease. Transgenic animals may be used for a variety of sophisticated studies on gene expression and function, including dosage effects and ectopic expression.

4.6 Understanding cardiovascular development

Development of human heart starts from a primordium in the cardiogenic plate, where angiogenic cell clusters coalesce to form two endocardial tubes, which later fuse together to form a single tube, subdivided into primordial heart chambers.

In the tubular heart, expression of most genes coding for contractile proteins shows either homogeneous expression, or a gradient along antero-posterior myocardial tube. At this stage, a peristaltoid contraction wave is observed, with a posterior-anterior pacemaker polarity.

Heart tube grows rapidly and bends upon itself, forming the bulboventricular loop. Septa begin to grow in atria, ventricle and bulbus cordis, thus forming the four heart chambers, pulmonary artery and aorta. Thus, five different functional segments are present: two fast-contracting segments, atria and ventricles (originated from the outer curvature of the primary heart tube) and three slow-conducting segments: inflow tract, atrioventricular canal and outflow tract. Ventricles at this stage show a trabeculated morphology. Eventually, an outer ventricular compact myocardial layer is formed, with a distinct pattern of expression. No ventricular conduction system is morphologically identifiable, athough a syncronous contraction wave, from apex to the anterior pole, may be observed.

Table 4.12: Some mouse genes relevant to development of the cardiovascular system, as shown by phenotypes corresponding to knock-out of selected genes. Developmental stages at which lethality is observed are reported in column 2 (from Koblizeck, 1999)

Gene	Lethal	Knock-out phenotype
Cytokines		
VEGF	E11	Impaired vasculogenesis and angiogenesis
Ang-1	E12	Reduced trabeculation, remodelling, pericyte recruitment
Neuregulin	E11	Reduced trabeculation
TGFβ1	E10.5	Variable defects during vasculogenesis
Receptors		
Flk1	E10	No endothelial differentiation and vasculogenesis
Flt1	E9.5	Disorganized vessels During vasculogenesis
ErbB2/4	<E11	Reduced trabeculation
Tie-1	E13.5	Oedema and hemorrhages
Tie-2	E10	Reduced trabeculation, perycite recruitment, remodelling, sprouting
TGFβRII	<E13.5	Defective vasculogenesis
Signalling		
B-Raf	<E13.5	Enlarged vessels, endothelial apoptosis
RasGAP	E10	Impaired remodelling, aberrant sprouting (dorsal aorta)
SOS1	E12	Hemorrhages, reduced trabeculation
Gα13	E10	Absence of tube formation (yolk sac), disorganized vessels (head)
Transcription		
TEL	E11	Defective angiogenesis (yolk sac)
LKLF	E13.5	Impaired tunica media formation and aneurysms

Transgenic mice have shown the presence of distinct transcriptional potentials in right and left atrial and ventricular components.

128

Ventricular conduction system derive from trabeculations, as suggested by expression patterns of genes coding for myosin light chain and myosin heavy chain isoforms, atrial natriuretic factor, GLN2 antigen, creatine-kinase isoforms and troponin isoforms (Franco, 1999).

Knock-out mice enabled to identify several genes relevant to development of the cardiovascular system. They include cytokines and their receptors, signalling molecules, transcription factors and extracellular matrix proteins (Tab.4.12). An extensive table of genes involved in cardiovascular morphogenesis was provided by Chin (1998).

Novel data are expected to come from application of DNA microarray technology to transgenic mice. Knock-out of single genes often induces upregulation of additional genes and dowregulation of others. Identification of such alterations should greatly help in unravelling functional relationships between genes contributing to a given phenotype. In mouse, cDNA microarrays were successfully applied in determining molecular phenotype in cardiac growth, development and response to injury (Sehl, 2000), and in induction and regression of experimental hypertrophy (Friddle, 2000).

SUMMARY In the last years, relevant progress was made in the identification of genes involved in inherited structural and functional diseases of the myocardium. All the four classical clinical entities (Hypetrophic cardiomyopathy, Dilated Cardiomyopathy, Arrhythmogenic Right Ventricular Cardiomyopathy and Restrictive Cardiomyopathy) resulted highly heterogeneous from genetic point of view. Actually, mutations in different genes were discovered, which cause such cardiomyopathies. Myocardiocyte normal performance is based on the integrity of different functional modules, as the energy production system, the contractile machinery, the complex of outer membrane-cytoskeleton and cell-to cell interactions, and so on. . Each of these modules relies on the function of several different proteins. Therefore a mutation in any gene encoding a protein involved in a module is expected to alter the function of the module itself.   ->

This view was recently summarized in the "final common pathway" hypothesis. Dilated cardiomyopathies seem to derive mostly from defective anchorage of sarcomere to cytoskeleton, hypertrophic cardiomyopathy are mostly due to defects in the contraction machinery and right ventricular cardiomyopathies might possibly result from defects in intercellular connections.

Also "pure" arrhythmic disorders are genetically heterogeneous. In these disorders, the involved functional module deals with the maintainance of correct concentration of ions across membranes. A genetic defect in any component of an ionic channel is expected to produce a pathogenic alteration in this compartment, manifested as arrhythmias of different type.

Congenital heart defects are also very heterogeneous. Most of them derive from mutations in genes active during early phases of development. Genetic dissection of developmentally abnormal phenotypes is conducted by aid of transgenic animals, in which specific genes are artificially kocked-out or targeted by mutations.

CHAPTER 5

INHERITED CARDIOVASCULAR DISORDERS

5.1 Structural defects of vessels

Previous chapter dealt with cardiac defects due to structural or functional alterations of myocardium. In this chapter, main vascular defects affecting the cardiac function will be considered, starting with structural defects due to intrinsic alteration of vessel wall.

Marfan's syndrome (autosomal dominant, OMIM 154700) is a disorder of the connective tissue, due to mutations of fibrillin (FBN1, mapped to 15q13.23). One of the most important clinical features of this disease is progressive dilation of the aortic root, due to reduced deposition of fibrillin in the vascular adventitia. Affected individuals show a consistently increased risk of aortic aneurysm and dissecation. As expected, wide phenotypic variability is observed, due to differences in individual genetic background and to environmental factors. Moreover fibrillin-1 genotype was found associated with aortic stiffness and disease severity, in patients with coronary artery disease (Medley, 2002).

Ehlers-Danlos syndrome (autosomal dominant, OMIM 130000) is due to mutation of the COL3A gene, mapped to 2q31 and encoding type III pro-collagen. Affected individuals show hyperelasticity of skin and connective tissue and hyperextensibility of joints. In most severe forms, mitral valve prolapse, aneurysm formation and even spontaneous rupture of large vessels may occur.

Fibromuscular dysplasia of arteries is an autosomal dominant disorder (OMIM 135580), manifested as arterial occlusive disease of children or young adults and producing hypertension, myocardial infarction or stroke. Association with hypertrophic cardiomyopathy was reported in some cases. Celiac and mesenteric arteries show a typical chain-of-beads appearance.

The above cited genetic diseases are rare. On the contrary, two cardiovascular disorders are very relevant in terms of morbidity and mortality: coronary artery disease and hypertension. Understanding genetic determination of these disorders is one of the major aims of present research.

5.2 Coronary atherosclerosis and myocardial infarction

Coronary Atherosclerotic Disease (CAD) is a major cause of morbidity and mortality in industrialized countries. In U.S., every year about 1,500,000 persons develop myocardial infarction (MI).

Several epidemiological studies identified, among CAD risk factors, a genetic predisposition to the disease.

In spite of a large wealth of studies, molecular pathophysiology of CAD is still not fully understood. Two different processes may be delineated: a) gradual development of obstructive atheriosclerotic lesions leading to stable angina; b) rapid progression of these lesions, leading to acute coronary syndromes.

According to present views, activation of vascular endothelium may cause a series of effects ending in mononuclear leukocytes recruitment into the vessel wall and subsequent release of cytokines and growth factors (Fig. 5.1).

These molecules would induce, directly or/and indirectly, smooth muscle cells migration and proliferation, along with alteration in the extracellular matrix.

On the other hand, activated smooth muscle cells would release molecules acting on other smooth muscle cells, on leukocytes and on platelets. Leukocytes seem to play a central role in atherogenesis. Monocyte-derived foam cells are a major component of atheromas. Moreover, white blood cells release growth factors (PDGF, bFGF) and cytokines (IL-1, TNF-α , IFN-γ and chemokines).

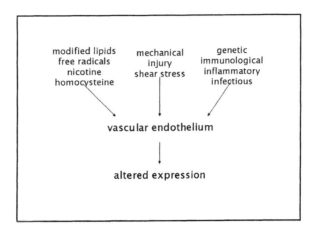

Figure 5.1 : Many different causes may induce altered endothelial response, leading to atherosclerosis.

CAD acute phase starts with the rupture of an atherosclerotic plaque; its exposure to blood would trigger the clot formation and propagation, leading to thrombosis.

It has been estimated that possibly over 400 genes are involved in lipoprotein metabolism, endothelial performance, inflammation and coagulation. Among them, probably the most investigated in the context of CAD are those involved in lipoprotein metabolism. Genetic investigations identified so far a small number of genes whose mutations underlie clinical phenotypes.

Familial Hypercholesterolemia (autosomal dominant, mapped to 19p13, OMIM 143890) is due to mutations in LDLR gene (Low-Density Lipoprotein Receptor). Individuals homozygous for LDLR mutations (prevalence 1/100,000) show clinical coronary atherosclerosis in the first or second decade of life, while heterozygotes (prevalence 1:500) develop coronary atherosclerosis in the fourth or fifth decade. It is interesting to notice that among survivors of myocardial infarction, frequency of heterozygotes for LDLR mutations is 1:20.

The disease has a worldwide distribution. Over 700 mutations (point mutations, deletions and splice mutations) were described so far in several human populations. Mutant LDL receptor shows reduced ability in removing apolipoprotein B (apoB) and apolipoprotein E (apoE) from bloodstream. Disease severity correlates with severity of mutations: those producing complete inactivation of LDL receptor cause premature atherosclerosis.

Familial Hypercholesterolemia, type 2 (autosomal recessive, mapped to 1p36-p35, OMIM 603813). Homozygotes show very elevated LDL cholesterol, tuberous and tendon xantomata and premature coronary atherosclerosis. The disease seems to be particularly frequent in Sardinia. Mutations were reported in a putative adaptor protein, named ARH (Autosomal Recessive Hypercholesterolemia). A recent study showed that small number, high frequency in the population and dispersed distribution of pathogenic variants are consistent with hypothesis that these mutations are ancient and were maintained in Sardinian population by geographical isolation (Arca, 2002)

Familial Hypercholesterolemia, type 3 (FH3, autosomal dominant, mapped to 1p34.1-p32, OMIM 603776) is characterized by selective increase of LDL particles in plasma, tendon and skin xantomas, acus corneae and premature mortality for cardiovascular complications. The involved gene is at the moment unknown.

Familial Defective Apolipoprotein B100 (FDB, autosomal dominant, mapped to 2q24, OMIM 107730) is a relatively common disease (prevalence 1:500, except in Finland where this disorder is rare). Clinical phenotype is similar to hypercholesterolemia. Mutations in gene apoB100 decrease affinity of apoB100 for LDL-receptor. It is interesting to note that over 99% of reported mutations correspond to a single aminoacid substitution (R3500Q). It has been reported that homozygosity for E2 isoform of Apo-E leads to atherosclerosis and premature cardiovascular disease, due to very high levels of cholesterol and of tryglycerides in VLDL fraction.

Also mutations in LPL (lipoprotein lipase) gene seem to increase risk for cardiovascular diseases, since their frequency was found higher among cardiovascular patients than among controls (Mailly, 1995). It is interesting that a peculiar mutation, which truncates the C-terminus of the protein, is protective, instead of pathogenic (Hokanson, 1997).

A polymorphism in the LPL gene, detected by HindIII digestion, revealed that H+/H+ genotype has a deleterious effect on lipid profile in presence of adverse environmental factors, such as cigarette smoking, while physical activity seems to reduce this effect (Senti, 2001).

Genotype-phenotype relationships are less clear for mutations of gene encoding apolipoprotein(a). The number of its "kringle" repeats inversely correlates to level of Lp(a), but pro-atherogenic effect of Lp(a) is strongly influenced by environmental factors.

Similarly, decreased level of High-Density-Lipoprotein (HDL) cholesterol , which is a known risk factor for cardiovascular disease, is under genetic control, but it may be induced by environmental factors, as sedentary habit and cigarette smoking.

Genome-wide linkage analyses were performed, aimed at identifying chromosomal regions hosting genes involved in atherosclerosis.

A genome-wide scan conducted in 99 families from Indo-Mauritian population (showing the highest prevalence in the world for coronary heart disease), identified a susceptibility locus on chromosome 16p13 (Francke, 2001). In a different study, evidence was obtained in favour of genes on chromosomes 4 and 5, influencing variation in the apolipoprotein A-II level, on chromosome 12, influencing variation in apolipoprotein A-I level, and on chromosome 17, influencing variation of total cholesterol/HDL-cholesterol ratio (Klos, 2001).

A comparable study, performed in 25 Finnish families, identified loci involved in low HDL-cholesterol level, mapped to chromosomes 8q23, 16q24.1.q24.2 and 20q13.11 (Soro, 2002).

Autosomal genome-wide scan was performed in sibships at high risk for hypertension, looking for coronary artery calcification loci. Two chromosomal regions (6p21.3 and 10q21.39 were identified, which could harbour genes associated with subclinical coronary atherosclerosis (Lange, 2002).

A whole genome scan, performed on 513 families, succeeded in identifying different loci involved in susceptibility to myocardial infarction and coronary artery disease. Elevated serum concentation of apolipoprotein (a) showed linkage with apolipoprotein (a) locus and with a novel locus on chromosome 1. Linkage with myocardial infarction and coronary artery disease was detected also for diabetes mellitus locus, on chromosome 6, for hypertension on chromosomes 1 and 6, for high-density and low-density lipoprotein cholesterol, on chromosomes 1 and 17, and for triglycerides concentations, on chromosome 9. But, the most interesting finding was the detection of significant linkage for a novel susceptibility locus, mapped to chromosome 14 (Broeckel, 2002).

It is important to note that differences in results among genome scan studies may partially derive from population differences. This is particularly true when dealing with hypercholesterolemia: it is known that this disease is mostly due to LDLR mutations in Iceland (Gudnason, 1997), to ApoB mutations in Switzerland (Miserez, 1994) and to FH3 mutations in South Asia (Khoo, 2000).

A different facet of genetic predisposition to atherosclerosis and coronary heart disease is the possibility that some individuals are genetically "resistant" to atherosclerosis, despite high cholesterol intake or elevated low-density lipoprotein cholesterol (LDL-C) levels.

The response to dietary cholesterol intake is mainly due to liver X receptor (LXR). Cholesterol absorption is affected also by Apo-E (Apolipoprotein-E), by SR-B1(scavenger receptor B1) and by ACAT-2 (acylcoenzyme cholesterol acyltransferase-2). It was shown that high activity of scavenger receptor in presence of adequate amounts of Apo-E might contribute to resistance to atherosclerosis. Interindividual genetic variability in these functions is possible. This interesting subject was reviewed by Stein (2002).

Also mutations in genes involved in endothelial performance, inflammation and coagulation may increase the risk for coronary artery disease and myocardial infarction.

Frequency of specific variants of marker genes, supposedly predisposing to CAD and MI, was investigated in cohorts of patients and controls, in order to assess their prognostic significance.

After ACE (Angiotensin Converting Enzyme, OMIM 106180) gene was cloned, a deletion in intron 16 was described (variant D= Deletion), not infrequent in the population. The normal allele (without deletion) was named I (Insertion). Since 50% of the total interindividual variability of plasma ACE concentration was apparently due to I/D polymorphism, allele D frequency was studied in different populations and cohorts of patients, in order to establish its value as predictor of risk for myocardial infarction. Since the first report by Cambien (1992), who found association between ACE polymorphism and CAD, hundreds of scientific reports were published. Progressively, original enthusiasm about having at hand a simple and potent predictor of risk for myocardial infarction gave place to more prudent conclusions (Singer, 1996). At the end, a study which compared 4,629 cases of myocardial infarction with 5,934 controls, concluded that ACE D/D genotype was observed in 29.4% of MI cases and in 27.6% of controls (risk ratio 1.10, 95% confidence interval 1.00-1.21). Moreover, meta-analysis performed on previously published studies established a risk ratio between 1.0 and 1.1 for myocardial infarction in homozygotes for D allele (Keavney, 2000). Definitely, ACE I/D polymorphism cannot be considered a potent predictor of myocardial infarction, as it was originally proposed.

Several additional gene variants were reported as possibly associated with increased or decreased risk for coronary artery disease and myocardial infarction (Tab. 5.1).

Table 5.1: Some gene variants reportedly associated with increased or decreased risk for coronary artery disease and myocardial infarction (see text).

OMIM	Gene	Variant	Risk
	Lipid metabolism		
143890	LDR	Many	Increased
505747	ARH	Many	Increased
107730	ApoB100	Arg3500Glu	Increased
107741	ApoE	Many	Increased
238600	LPL	Asn291Ser	Increased
		Ser447stop	Decreased
	Blood pressure		
106150	AGT (Angiotensinogen)	Thr174Met	Increased
		Met235Thr	Increased
	Blood coagulation		
188040	THBD (Thrombomodulin)	Ala455Val	Increased
		1bpIns1689T	Increased
264900	F7 (Clotting Factor VII)	10bpIns-323	Decreased
		Arg353Gln	Decreased
134570	F13 (Clotting Factor XIII)	Val34Leu	Decreased

For instance, M allele of polymorphism T174M in gene encoding angiotensinogen was found associated with coronary atherosclerosis (Spiridonova, 2002) and a different polymorphism (M235T) of the same gene was also identified as associated with myocardial infarction (Fernandez-Arcas, 2001; Olivieri, 2001).

Among genes involved in the coagulation process, Thrombomodulin (THBD, OMIM 188040) polymorphic variants (Ala 25Thr; 1-bp ins, 1689T; Ala455Val) were reportedly associated with acute MI. It was observed that carrying Val allele of polymorphism Ala455Val increased risk of CAD by 6-fold in African-Americans but not significantly in Caucasians (Wu, 2001).

Risk-alleles for MI were detected in polymorphisms of genes GP Ib and GI?VI, encoding products which play crucial roles in initial adhesion of platelets to collagen, during formation of coronary thrombus (Croft, 2001; Mikkelsson, 2001).

On the other hand, variants of Factor VII (OMIM 227500), associated to decreased susceptibility to myocardial infarction, were reported (Girelli, 2000).

Inflammation is a prominent mechanism in pathogenesis of atherosclerosis and coronary thrombosis. A number of association studies were performed on following candidate marker genes: TNFs (tumour necrosis factor alpha and beta), TGFs (Transforming Growth Factors beta 1 and 2, IL (Interleukin 1), IL 1ra (Interleukin 1 receptor antagonist), CID 14 (receptor for lipopolysaccharide) P-Selectin, E-Selectin and PECAM-1(Platelet Endothelial Cell Adesion Molecule). Results were conflicting, as reported by a a recent review (Andreotti, 2002).

A few years ago, association between cardiovascular diseases and heterozygosity for the major mutation (C282Y) in HFE gene, involved in haemochromatosis, was suggested (critically reviewed by Sullivan, 1999). A recent study performed on two large case-control studies (ECTIM and GENIC) provided no consistent evidence supporting the hypothesis of association (Hetet, 2001).

In conclusion, many different gene variants possibly contribute to risk of developing MI; however, if we except the small number of cases affected with genetic alterations of lipid metabolism, none of the novel predictors based on DNA analysis seem potent enough to surmount "classical" predictors, i.e. age, family history of premature CAD/MI, HDL (<40mg/dl), hypertension (> 140/90 mmHg), diabetes mellitus.

Probably, this situation will change in the near future, when additonal DNA tests will be available, based on better understanding of molecular pathogenesis and on results from ongoing association studies.

The ACE story told us that association studies need very large numbers before reaching conclusions about predictive value of a DNA variant. Untimely enthusiasms not only raise false expectations, but risk introducing in medical practice tests with doubtful predictive value.

5.3 Genetics of hypertension

Blood pressure values are normally distributed among individuals of a given human population, thus indicating the multifactorial determination of such phenotype. It has been estimated that about 30% of observed inter-individual variability in blood pressure is due to genetic determination (Kaplan, 1998).

Hypertension is defined with reference to a threshold value (140/90 mmHg), which represents the limit beyond which risk for cardiovascular affections significantly increases.

Hypertension affects about 20% of people living in industrialized countries and significantly contributes to morbidity and mortality. In fact, abnormally high blood pressure is involved, as primary cause or as complicating factor, in different cardiovascular diseases, from myocardial infarction, to stroke and to renal failure.

In considering genetic determination of hypertension we should distinguish a limited number of rare hypertensive diseases showing mendelian inheritance (Tab. 5.2), from the more general problem of genetic predisposition to hypertension (Kroon, 2001).

Table 5.2: Mendelian hypertensive disorders (see text for details)

Disease	Gene	OMIM
Glucocorticoid-Remediable Aldosteronism (GRA)	CYP11B2	103900
Apparent Mineralocorticoid Excess syndrome (AME)	HSD11B2	218030
Liddle syndrome	SCNN1B	177200
,, ,,	SCNN1G	,,
Gordon's syndrome	WNK4	145260
,, ,,	WNK1	,,
,, ,,	?	,,
Dominant, early onset hypertension, exacerbated by pregnancy	NR3C2	600983
Adrenal Hyperplasia syndrome	CYP17	202110
Bardet-Biedl syndrome BBS2	MKKS2	606151
Bardet-Biedl syndrome BBS4	MKKS4	600374

Glucocorticoid-remediable Aldosteronism (GRA, autosomal dominant mapped to 8q21; OMIM 103900) is due to the presence of an abnormal gene, resulting from the fusion of part of gene CYP11B2 with part of gene CYP11B1. CYP11B1 encodes a steroid 11β-hydroxylase, which catalyzes last step of cortisol biosynthesis; CYP11B2 is a related gene, coding for a protein showing 11β-hydroxylase, 18-hydroxylase and 18-oxydase activities. Unequal crossing-over involving the two genes generated the "fusion gene".

In GRA, hypertension is manifested since early adult age. It is caused by excessive secretion of aldosterone, which, in turn, increases salt and water retention. There is an increased risk of cerebral hemorrages.

A simple DNA test is available to detect the presence of the abnormal gene (MacConnachie, 1998), thus avoiding biochemical characterization of the phenotype.

Apparent Mineralocorticoid Excess syndrome (AME, autosomal recessive, mapped to 16q22; OMIM 218030), is due to mutation in gene coding for 11-β-hydroxysteroid dehydrogenase, isoform 2 (HSD11B2). Several mutations in different human populations were reported in the literature. Heterozygotes for the pathogenic mutations are phenotypically normal, but they may show subtle defects in cortisol metabolism.

HSD11B2 catalyzed the transformation of cortisol to cortisone (which is unable to stimulate the mineralcorticoid receptor in the distal convoluted tubule of the kidney). In AME, mutant enzyme hinders conversion of cortisol to cortisone; the excess of cortisol hyperstimulates the receptor and, consequently, produces hypertension.

Liddle syndrome (autosomal dominant, mapped to 16p13-p12, OMIM 177200) is due to constitutive activation of renal epithelium sodium channel, due to mutation in either beta (SCNN1B) or gamma (SCNN1G) subunit. The disease is characterized by early-onset and frequently severe hypertension, associated with hypokalaemic alkalosis, low plasma renin activity and low aldosterone level.

Several mutations in SCNN1B and in SCNN1G were reported: missense mutations, stop codons and frame-shifts mutations generated by small deletions or insertions. All mutations increase activity of the altered subunit and, consequently, increase reabsortion of sodium in the distal convoluted tubule.

Gordon's syndrome (also named Pseudohypoaldosteronism, type II, PHA2; autosomal dominant, OMIM 145260) is caused by mutations in different genes: WNK4 (mapped to 17q21, OMIM 601844), WNK1 (mapped to 12p, OMIM 605232) and in a still unknown gene mapped to 1q31-q42. The syndrome, characterized by hypertensive hyperkalaemia, was reported in different human populations. Missense mutations were detected in WNK4 (PHAIIB), while in WNK1 (PHAIIC) an intragenic deletion was reported, but present data are far from being conclusive.

An autosomal dominant form of early-onset hypertension, with severe exacerbation in pregnancy (OMIM 600983) was described, due to mutation of the mineralocorticoid receptor NR3C2 (Geller, 2000).

Hypertension is an important component of the disease phenotype in Adrenal Hyperplasia V syndrome (autosomal recessive mapped to 10q24.3; OMIM 202110), due to mutations of different type (nucleotide deletions, duplications or substitutions) in CYP17 gene, encoding 17-α-hydroxylase, and in Bardet-Biedl syndrome (BBS, OMIM 209900). In BBS type 2 (autosomal recessive mapped to 16q21, OMIM 606151) and in BBS4 (autosomal recessive mapped to 15q22.3-q23, OMIM 600374) mutations were detected in genes belonging to the MKKS family. Proteins encoded by BBSs genes show sequence homology to the alpha unit of a bacterial chaperonin. Several different mutations were reported in BSS patients.

As far as predisposition to hypertension is concerned, the investigational approach is similar to that adopted for searching genetic predictors of coronary artery disease and myocardial infarction.

Possible association with hypertension was investigated by DNA polymorphisms in genes involved in three different functional modules: renin-angiotensin system, system regulating ions exchanges at the level of renal tubule, and sympathetic nervous system.

Renin-angiotensinogen system is well known (Fig. 5.2): a lowering of blood pressure stimulates the kidney to secrete renin, which cleaves angiotensin from angiotensinogen. Angiotensin is then converted into Angiotensin II.

Since Angiotensin represents the key molecule in raising blood pressure, attention of several investigators focussed on possible polymorphisms in genes encoding proteins involved in production of functional angiotensin.

Association of a polymorphic variant (Met235Thr) of Angiotensinogen (AGT) gene, with hypertension was reported since 1992 (Jeunemaitre, 1992); soon later, association of a different variant of the same gene (Thr174Met) with pre-eclampsia was reported (Ward, 1993). An additional variant, associated with hypertension, was detected in the proximal part of the promoter of AGT gene (Inoue,1997), probably affecting the basal rate of transcription in vivo.

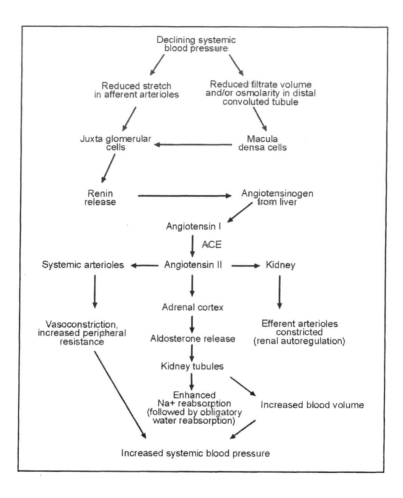

Figure 5.2 : An overwiew on blood pressure regulation

In spite of several reports in agreement with early findings, a European study failed to confirm significant association between AGT variants and hypertension (Brand, 1998).

As shown in Fig. 5.2, ACE (Angiotensin Converting Enzyme) plays a key role in the renin-angiotensin system. Its intronic I/D polymorphism was mentioned earlier in this chapter, with reference to its claimed predictory value for MI. Data regarding a possible association with renal disease are controversial (Taal, 2000), but D variant could be associated with atheromatous renal artery disease (Olivieri, 2002).

A DNA polymorphism (A1166C) in gene encoding angiotensin receptor II type 1 was detected and associated with hypertension and aortic stiffness (Bonnardeaux, 1994; Benetos, 1995). The presence of allele C seems to determine increased sensitivity to Angiotensin II (Spiering, 2000); this behaviour was observed also in isolated human arteries obtained from patients undergoing coronary artery bypass grafting (Van Geel, 2000).

A series of DNA polymorphisms so far reportedly associated with hypertension is shown in Tab. 5.3.

Table 5.3: Some gene variants reportedly associated with hypertension (see text for details).

OMIM	Gene	Variant
	Renin-angiotensin system	
106150	AGT (Angiotensinogen)	Thr174Met
	"	Met235Thr
	"	G-6A
106180	ACE (Angiotensin-converting-enzyme)	D
	AT1R (AngiotensinIII receptor)	A1166C
	CYP11B2 (Aldosterone synthase)	C-344T
	Renal tubule function	
	ADDU1 (Adducin 1)	Gly460TRP
	GNB3 (G protein β3)	825T
	Sympathetic nervous system	
	ADRB2 (β2 adrenergic receptor)	Arg16Gly

Detection of a polymorphism (C-344T) in the regulatory region of CYP11B2 gene (aldosterone synthase) raised strong interest, since aldosterone synthase is known to be involved in hypertension. Despite the fact that T allele was found more frequently among hypertensive patients than among controls, it is still debated if C-344T really corresponds to a functional variant of the gene (Kroon, 2001).

Hypertension may develop because of defects at the level of renal tubule. A polymorphism (Gly460Trp) in gene coding for Adducin 1 (ADDU1) was described, associated with increased tubular sodium reabsorption, by possible interaction with Na+K+ ATPase (Ferrandi, 1997). Although contradictory results were obtained in the Japanese population (Kato, 1998), the association seems confirmed among Europeans (Kroon, 2001).

A DNA polymorphism (C825T) was discovered also in gene GNB3, coding for a subunit of the regulatory protein of the Na+H+exchanger. The nucleotide substitution cause an increase in the activity of the subunit. The association between this variant and hypertension was suggested (Poch, 2000), but no conclusive evidence was produced so far.

Finally, possible polymorphisms in genes involved in blood pressure regulation by sympathetic nervous system were sought.

Actually, association was detected between polymorphisms of α2-and β2 adrenergic receptor (Sevetkey, 1996; Kotanko, 1997; Bray, 2000). The variant Arg16Gly of ADRB2 (Adrenoreceptor beta-2) gene induces excessive agonist-mediated downregulation of the receptor, which increases peripheral vascular resistance and, hence, blood pressure.

Data here reported on associations between DNA polymorphisms and hypertension or CAD and MI witnesses important attempts in the identification of inherited determinants predisposing to the development of such diseases.

These data resulted mostly from a "candidate-gene approach": polymorphisms were sought in genes certainly or suspectedly involved in a biochemical step or pathway related to the considered disease. However, our present knowledge of cell biology and physiology is incomplete, thus several good candidate genes might have escaped consideration. The alternative approach, genome-wide scan, appears unbiased from this point of view, but in reality it suffers from different biases.

Results of a series of genome-wide scan studies, performed in the last few years, are summarized in Tab. 5.4. The overall picture gives the impression of a still undefined frame. Independent studies are mostly discordant and show rare overlaps of candidate chromosomal regions. Apparently, over fifteen different chromosomes possibly host genes involved in determination of blood pressure.

Table 5.4 : Results of different studies attempting to identify, by genome-wide scans, genetic factors affecting blood pressure (see text).

Author	Year	Chromosomal Regions
Systolic and diastolic blood pressure		
Hsueh	2000	2q31-q34
Zhu	2001	2q14-q23
Lange	2002	6p21.3, 10q21.3
Systolic blood pressure		
Krushkal	1999	2p22.1-p21, 5q33.3-q34, 6q23.1-q24.1, 15q25.1.q26.1
Pankow	2000	18q
Levy	2000	17
Rice	2000	1p, 2p, 5p, 7q, 8q, 19p
Diastolic blood pressure		
Levy	2000	17, 18
Perola	2000	AT1
Quantitative Trait Loci (QTLs)		
Atwood	2001	2,18, 21
Harrap	2002	1,4,16,X
Pre-eclampsia		
Arngrimsson	1999	2p13
Lachmeijer	2001	3p, 12q, 15q

Disagreement between results might be ascribed to different causes. The above-cited studies were performed in different populations: it is possible, but unproven, that variants of genes affecting blood pressure are the same in different and geographically distant populations. Geographical and historical factors might have produced differences not only between the considered samples, but also between sub-groups of the same population. Particularly interesting in this respect are the two studies on pre-eclampsia, performed on Icelandic (Arngrimssom, 1999) and on Dutch (Lachmeijer, 2001) population. On the basis of the clear definition of clinical phenotype and of the common European origin of the two populations, a concordance in results was expected. On the contrary, the Dutch study failed to confirm the results obtained in Icelandic population.

Different problems may be encountered when dealing with a sample from a population of recent genetic admixture: in such cases stratification may be controlled with great difficulty.

As far as methodology is concerned, we should recall that linkage analysis is a very conservative method, developed for localizing genes involved in determination of monogenic phenotypes. In a genome-wide linkage analysis for identifying genes involved in polygenic-multifactorial phenotype, it is highly improbable to obtain lod scores above 3, since several genes are involved and each one of them is expected to have a moderate effect on phenotype. On the other hand, if level of significance is lowered, i.e. by accepting lod scores below 3.0, the background noise, i.e. number of false positive and false negative "signals", will increase, thus possibly producing variable results in different studies.

All the above-cited investigations were based on the analysis of 350 to 450 markers, while a "dense" genome scan usually includes about 800 markers. In a genome scan using a "loose" grid of markers and applied to the search of genes involved in a polygenic phenotype, the *a priori* probability of detecting linkage at a given locus is very low, since it is improbable that: 1) a single gene shows a major effect on phenotype; 2) this gene lies close to one of the markers used for the genome scan .

Genome-wide scans are expensive: analyzing 300 sib pairs for 700 markers means to perform 420,000 individual PCR reactions....just to start with. Therefore, in each study a compromise is made between number of individuals to be genotyped and number of markers. Both the number of markers and sample size are really critical; moreover, a relatively small sample size would increase the adverse effect of possible and unrecognized stratification.

At this point it should be clear that localizing and identifying genes involved in common chronic diseases is really a formidable challenge.

Recent and present studies should be still considered as pilot studies. Experience gained by present investigations will greatly help in designing subsequent searches. For instance, studies on large pedigrees already demonstrated to be more powerful than those on relative pairs and multipoint variance-components linkage analysis (Rice, 2000; Rankinen, 2001) appeared to be an interesting approach.

A comprehensive review on genetics of hypertension, with particular reference to the development of association and linkage studies was produced by Doris (2002).

5.4 Understanding hypertension through animal models

Transgenic and knock-out animals represent the most powerful research tool for genetic dissection of complex phenotypes. Transgenic and knock-out mice were produced for analyzing the role of different genes involved in renin-angiotensin system or in other systems known to regulate vascular tone and/or electrolyte and fluid homeostasis (Cvetkovic, 2000).

A series of genes shown to be involved in determination of blood pressure by targeted deletion is shown in Tab. 5.5.

On the other hand, a mouse model of pre-eclampsia was obtained simply by breeding, in a mouse strain showing mildly elevated blood pressure (Davisson, 2002).

Spontaneous hypertensive rat (SHR) is the most widely studied animal model of essential hypertension. A few years ago, transfer of one segment of chromosome 8 from a normotensive strain in a SHR genetic background resulted in a substantial reduction in systolic and diastolic blood pressure

(Kren,1997). More recently, gene(s) responsible for a wide spectrum of cardiovascular risk factors were reported to map to a limited segment of the centromeric region of rat chromosome 4; a spontaneous deletion in gene Cd36, encoding a fatty acid transporter and located within the above region, was found linked to transmission of insulin resistance, defective fatty acid metabolism and increased blood pressure (Pravenec, 2000).

Rat X syndrome includes hypertension, dyslipidemia, impaired glucose tolerance, obesity and coronary artery disease. A major QTL for glucose metabolism was detected on chromosome 3, other QTLs for obesity and body weight on chromosome 1 and 5, and determinants for dyslipidemia on chromosomes 4 and 17 (Kovacs, 2000).

Table 5.5 : Targeted gene deletions in mice, affecting blood pressure.

Gene	Code
Angiotensin type 2 receptor	Agtr2
Apolipoprotein E	ApoE
Bradykinin receptor type 2	Bdkrb2
Calcium-dependent K+ channel β1sub	Kcnmb1
Cytochrome p450 monoxygenase 4A14	Cyp41a14
Dopamine receptor	Drd3
Dopamine regulated phophoprotein	Ppp1r1b
Endothelial nitric oxide	Nos3
Heme oxygenase	Hmox1
11-β-Hydroxysteroid dehydrogenase II	Hsd11b2
Insulin receptor substrate	Irs1
Natriuretic peptide receptor	Npr1
Protein tyrosine phosphatase type 0	Ptpr0

More recently, two blood pressure QTLs were mapped on chromosome 10 in Dahl rats (Sivo, 2002)

Comparative genomics of mammals is quickly progressing. The complete DNA sequence of mouse genome will be available soon and rat genome is now being explored.

As soon as the complete mouse genome is available, it will be possible to establish firm correspondences between human and mouse genes. At this point, genetic investigations on mice (from expression profiling to genome-wide linkage analyses) will produce information directly related to human physiology in health and disease. It is difficult to forecast how much this revolution would affect medical practice, but definitely it will occur very soon.

SUMMARY Beside inherited defects of myocardial cells, other genetic alterations may affect the cardiovascular system. Some of them are inherited as mendelian traits, like Marfan's syndrome or Fibromuscular dysplasia of arteries, while others, like coronary atherosclerosis and hypertension are multifactorial disorders, due to combination of alterations in several genes and to environmental effects. Present research aims at identifying genes involved in these multifactorial disease, since identification of susceptibility genes may help in defining individual risk, possibly through genetic tests.

So far, a small number of rare genetic diseases of lipid metabolism have been described, associated with increased risk for coronary artery disease and myocardial infarction, but none of the novel proposed predictors, based on DNA analyses, proved to be potent enough to surmount classical predictors still used in clinical practice.

Possible associations between DNA variants and hypertension were investigated by candidate-gene approach, i.e. by testing genes certainly or suspectedly involved in a biochemical step or pathway related to the disease.

More recently, genome-wide scan was applied, in order to test association with each of many DNA markers scattered along human chromosomes. No conclusive results were obtained, but evidence was reached pointing at some chromosomal localizations.

The availability of complete sequence of mouse genome enables comparative studies with human genome.

Genetic investigation on mice, from linkage studies to expression profiling, will soon produce data which will help in understanding human physiology in health and disease, including genetic predisposition to hypertension or to other cardiovascular disorders.

Several rodent models of hypertension already produced interesting data on chromosomal localization of genes involved in such disease

CHAPTER 6

GENETICS AND GENOMICS APPLIED TO DIAGNOSIS AND THERAPY

6.1 Growing interest for genetic tests

Since the time of pioneering studies on hemoglobin mutations causing sickle-cell anemia it was clear that DNA analysis could enable the detection of pathogenic variations in disease genes.

The methodological revolution brought by PCR and by automated DNA sequencing both accelerated the discovery of disease genes and provided many laboratories with the possibility of detecting pathogenic mutations. At the beginning, DNA testing was exclusively addressed to prenatal diagnosis of very severe genetic diseases, such as sickle-cell anemia, thalassemia, cystic fibrosis and Duchenne muscular dystrophy. As soon as the first catalogue of polymorphic DNA markers was released in 1992 by Genethon, the possibility of detecting "at-risk" alleles by analysis of flanking polymorphic markers became feasible and paved the way to DNA testing even for diseases where the disease locus was established, but the involved gene was still unknown.

In the last ten years an incredible increase of knowledge on human genome took place, accompanied by an unprecedented popularization of genetic discoveries. Words as *genome, genes* and *genetic tests* became very familiar to the general public, not only through TV educational programs, but more often through TV news and newspapers. People got the message that, since all diseases have a genetic component, it is possible to discover individual predisposition to diseases, by a simple DNA test. Soon, the idea of having at hand "absolute" tests for detecting the presence of severe diseases, much before their clinical manifestation, gained popularity in US and in other industrialized countries; the number of performed genetic tests increased there year by year, causing some concern among geneticists and genetic counsellers.

The Task Force on Genetic Testing, a joint Department of Energy and National Institutes of Health working group, defined as "genetic testing" any procedure of analysis of human DNA, RNA, chromosomes, proteins and metabolites, able to establish a diagnosis of a genetic disease, to predict risk of developing an inheritable disorder and to identify carriers of mutations related to such affections. Prenatal tests, newborn screening, carrier screening and testing in families with a history of a genetic disorders are all considered an integral part of genetic testing.

Presently, clinical genetic testing is available for over 900 diseases, but for about 350 of them tests are still performed only in research laboratories as part of their investigations. Most simple DNA tests cost about $200 each, while more sophisticated tests may require over $3,000.

The general public believes that genetic tests, are simple and absolutely precise, because they are based on DNA. In reality, the problem of DNA tests is more complicated than generally perceived, as we will see in this Chapter.

6.2 Purposes and methods of genetic testing

Genetic tests are used for different purposes:

a) Preimplantation diagnosis, performed after *in vitro* fertilization, in order to detect the eventual presence of a genetic defect in an embryo, before artificial implantation. For this purpose, DNA analysis of a single blastomere is currently used.

b) Prenatal diagnosis, usually performed at 12-14 weeks of gestation, by chorionic villus sampling and subsequent DNA analysis, in order to detect a genetic defect in the developing fetus.

c) <u>Newborn screening</u>, aiming at early detection of babies affected with treatable genetic diseases; traditional methods, as PKU screening, are still widely used, but novel DNA technologies are ahead.

d) <u>Carrier testing</u>: this approach aims at detecting heterozygous carriers in specific geographical areas showing high incidence of a severe disease. For instance, in Sardinia, where frequency of heterozygotes for beta-thalassemia is very high, local health authority offered to all spouses free DNA testing for the most common beta-thalassemia mutation. In this way, couples carrying the pathogenic mutation could be detected and early prenatal diagnosis could be offered to them.

e) <u>Diagnostic DNA testing</u>: for some genetic diseases a precise diagnosis may be difficult, when based only on clinical evidences. DNA test may greatly help in these cases and in resolving genetic heterogeneity.

f) <u>Pre-symptomatic DNA testing</u>: in this case DNA analysis is performed with the aim of detecting a pathogenic mutation in an apparently healthy individual. For some diseases, like Huntington Chorea, risk associated with presence of the mutant allele is firmy established; on the contrary, in most genetic diseases data are still insufficient to produce a precise risk estimation. Situation is even worst in cases of *predictive* DNA testing applied to mutation(s) producing a small increase of risk to develop a given disease. In these instances, prediction is often inaccurate.

The word "DNA test" applies to a series of different methods sharing in common the object of the analysis, DNA, and the aim, direct or indirect, of detecting a pathogenic variation in one gene.

Let's consider different situations, with respect to application of DNA tests to inherited diseases which clinical phenotype was already clearly defined.

<u>Mendelian inheritance, but no information available on the involved gene nor on its chromosomal location</u>. This is an unfavourable situation (no DNA test is applicable), but the progress of knowledge on human genome is likely

156

to provide in the near future the missing information and quickly open the way to DNA testing.

Mendelian inheritance, but information available only on chromosomal location. If the patient is an isolated case, no DNA test is applicable. On the contrary, if a dominant disease runs in a family, it is possible to analyze a series of polymorphic DNA markers (VNTRs or SNPs) located within the "critical region" where the unknown gene is hidden and to follow the segregation of haplotypes in the family, in order to identify the "at-risk" haplotype associated with the presence of the disease.

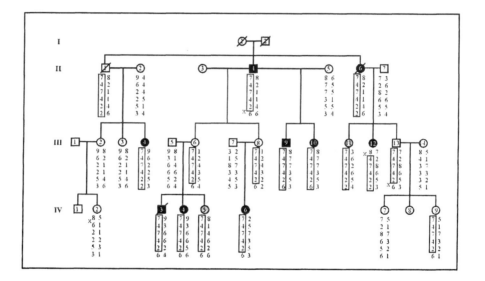

Figure 6.1: A family in which an autosomal dominant disease is transmitted associated with a given (boxed) haplotype. The DNA analysis of relatives of affected cases may detect that some individuals (III,6; III,8; III,13; IV,9) carry the "at-risk" haplotype and therefore might develop the disease.

Each family has his own at-risk haplotype running through generations. Once the risk-haplotype would have been identified, it is possible to test an individual DNA for the presence of such haplotype (Fig. 6.1), for pre-symptomatic diagnosis.

If the disease is inherited as recessive trait, again the analysis would reveal the at-risk haplotype, carried in homozygosis by the affected individuals.

The success of the investigation strongly depends on the size of the family, on the availability of DNA from family members and on the informativity of selected polymorphic DNA markers. The higher the number of closely spaced polymorphic markers, the higher will be the probability of detecting eventual recombinations within the critical region, which could adversely affect risk prediction. In case DNA markers are loosely spaced, the possibility of missing double recombinants must always be considered.

Mendelian inheritance and full information available on the involved gene. This is the most favourable situation, since, in principle, the knowledge of the involved gene should enable detection of any possible mutation in its DNA sequence.

In reality, only detection of nucleotide substitution in coding sequences is a relatively easy task, although some difficulty may arise from the large size of a gene or from high number of its exons.

Detection of some mutations (e.g. heterozygous deletions) may require a specific experimental approach; other mutations (e.g. mutation in cryptic slicing sites, within introns) can be detected only by analyzing the entire genomic sequence (exons and introns) of the considered gene, or by cDNA sequencing. Mutations in regulatory sequences can be detected with even more difficulty: nucleotide variation is frequent in intragenic and in extragenic non-coding sequences, thus making it difficult to discriminate between "normal" and "abnormal" variation.

The rate of detection of nucleotide substitutions reaches 100% only when direct DNA sequencing is applied. Any other method adopted for mutation screening shows a lower detection rate. Instrumental errors and mistakes in interpretation of results may also occur in DNA investigations, as in any other laboratory procedure.

Some genes show a prevalent type of mutations (e.g. intragenic deletions rather than nucleotide substitutions); therefore, standard procedures for detecting mutations may differ from gene to gene.

Only a few genes show mutational hot-spots or a relatively small number of "common" mutations, thus simplifying the investigation; in the majority of cases, the search for a causative mutation in a given gene is a difficult work, usually consisting in a multi-step process (Tab. 6.1).

Table 6.1: Different steps in detection of a causative mutation in a given gene, listed in order of priority of investigation

	Type of mutation	Method
1	Nucleotide change in coding sequence	DHPLC, DNA sequencing
2	Intragenic deletions or duplications	Southern blot
3	Activation of a cryptic splicing site	cDNA sequencing
4	Regulatory mutation	Northern blot/DNA sequencing

Once a mutation would be detected, its role in causing the disease phenotype should be defined, unless the specific mutation has already been described. The pathogenic role of a newly detected mutation is immediately evident only when a stop codon, disruption of the reading frame or alteration of the correct series of exons is produced. On the contrary, to prove pathogenicity of missense mutations may be problematic, since possibility that the detected variation is non-pathogenic cannot be immediately ruled out (see Chapter 3, section 3.6).

A causative mutation detected in a patient becomes "diagnostic" for additional members of the same family; moreover, the knowledge that a given mutation produced a given clinical phenotype may be very useful when other patients and families are analyzed, in any situation of genetic testing.

For some genes, a list of described mutations is available in Mutation Databases (see Appendix I), thus facilitating the investigation.

Current methodological approach for detecting a mutation in a given gene is DHPLC analysis (low-cost and high detection rate), followed by DNA sequence of the DNA segment which showed abnormal elution pattern (see Chapter 3, Section 3.5).

When mutation screening is performed on a patient's DNA for diagnostic purposes, detection of a causative mutation is always diagnostic, while a negative result doesn't necessarily mean that the patients is affected with a different disease: it simply means that the mutation has not been found. Genetic heterogencity and the possibility of phenocopies should always be considered.

Mitochondrial DNA inheritance. The search for mutations in mitochondrial DNA includes analysis of specific mutations in mtDNA, screening for mtDNA deletions, and screening the entire (16.6 kb) mtDNA for point mutations. Investigation involves the same methods and problems encountered in mutation detection in nuclear DNA. A very important point in mtDNA testing is the impossibility of predicting severity of clinical phenotypes in persons who inherited a mutant mtDNA, because of heteroplasmy (see Chapter 2, section 2.8).

Multifactorial inheritance. As seen in Chapter 2, Section 2.9, multifactorial diseases are due to a mix of genetic and environmental determinants. Usually, several genes contribute to phenotype, each one with a relatively small effect. Analytical methods for such conditions should imply simultaneous detection of genetic variants in several genes. Therefore they will probably develop in the near future from present DNA-chip technology.

Genetic tests predictive of multifactorial cardiovascular disorders are still in an early phase of development; results reported in the literature on this subject should be taken as preliminary data, unless sensitivity (% of true positives detected among affected individuals tested), specificity (% of true negatives among unaffected individuals tested), positive predictive value (% of true positives among positive tests) and negative predictive value (% of true negatives among negative tests) were established. Clinical validity (i.e. test's accuracy in identifying or predicting a given disease) and clinical utility (i.e. usefulness of the test for the individual being tested) of a proposed test should be considered before introduction in clinical practice. In this respect, DNA tests are not different from biochemical tests.

6.3 Novel genetic tests

Presently, interest of doctors and patients is focused on possible introduction in clinical practice of DNA tests which could provide reliable prediction of risk of developing a given inherited disease.

The problem is particularly relevant in Cardiology, due to high prevalence of coronary atherosclerotic disease and myocardial infarction in the general population. On one side, adult men and women, worried about their biological destiny, ask for simple and precise predictors and believe that genetic analyses are the wanted "ultimate" test; on the other side, physicians are permanently under conflicting pressures of maintaining a prudent attitude toward novel tests with still unproved efficiency and of avoiding risk of malpractice suits because they didn't suggest genetic testing to their patients.

According to our present knowledge, in multifactorial diseases a variation in one or more of several genes may be necessary, but not sufficient to cause the disease. Therefore any prediction becomes problematic: even if we knew all genes contributing to determination of a given multifactorial disease and we had detected and identified all variants of these genes in the given proband, we couldn't establish a *precise* risk for him, due to the ignorance of the environmental factors which acted on the considered individual. At least in the near future, genetic diagnosis might hardly become a robust and potent predictor of clinical phenotypes, although it might become an useful ancillary tool to evaluate individual susceptibility . Actually the detection of "risky" variants in a given individual might contribute to assess his personal situation (see later in this chapter), provided that extensive information is available on risk associated with each variant, and with presence of different variants in the same genotype.

The present dilemma (test or not to test?) may be possibly solved by informing the consultant about the predictive power of available DNA tests. Present genetic tests may add only a small fraction to the individual risk value calculated on the ground of clinical information and biochemical data.

The problem of false positives is probably restricted to possible adverse psychological effects of the knowledge of carrying a "risky" genotype, unless a drug with potentially adverse effects would be administered as a preventive treatment. Some persons which resulted positive to the test may feel "sentenced" and change plans for their life; some other might become very depressed or may become anxious and ask for hyper-medicalization. On the other hand, perception of the existence of an increased risk of developing a disease might persuade a person with a positive DNA test to adopt a more healthy lifestyle. We might be tempted to conclude rather cynically that, in this case, the communication of a non-existing risk might result, at the end, beneficial; however we should remember that everyone has the right to know the truth about his disease.

A more serious problem arises from the fraction of false negatives which will develop a disease or which will eventually encounter sudden death, in spite of negative results of their genetic tests. No lawsuits on this specific matter were brought yet to the Courts, at least to my knowledge.

Coming to the future of tests, as reported in Chapter 2, section 1, probably DNA microchip and cDNA array technology will be applied relatively soon to clinical diagnosis. It is possible that in the future these methods could enable simultaneous detection of mutations in a relevant number of genes involved in mendelian diseases, or in genes involved in multifactorial diseases. We may also envisage further technological advancements, prompted by development of proteomics.

Also for these innovative methods, adequate evaluation of their analytical validity, clinical validity and clinical utility will be necessary before introduction in clinical practice.

6.4 Genetic risk assessment

When dealing with inherited diseases, risk assessment concerns two different aspects: a) probability that a given individual (proband) would develop a given disease, and b) probability that additional case(s) could occur in the index case family, in the present or in the future generation(s)

In both instances, a careful analysis of the family history is the first and most important step of the investigation.

Proband has no affected relatives in the present or past three generations: his/her risk to develop the considered inherited disease equals the mutation rate, if the pathogenic trait is inherited as autosomal dominant, and roughly corresponds to incidence rate of the disease, if the trait is inherited as autosomal recessive. In a X-linked recessive disease, if the proband is a male, probability of manifestation in the absence of a positive family history will roughly equal mutation rate. If the proband is a female, the likelihood of manifestation in the absence of positive family history corresponds to the prevalence rate of the affected female phenotype in the general population.

Proband has a positive family history and the pattern of inheritance of the disease is known: the *a priori* probability of having inherited the genotype determining the manifestation of the disease may be computed simply by application of probability laws to segregation of chromosomes in each generation. In Fig. 6.2 a family tree is reported, showing the inheritance of an autosomal dominant disease, manifesting its effects after 35 years of age.

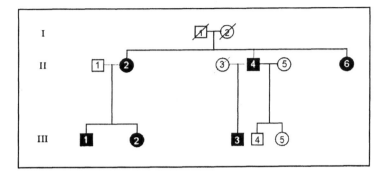

Figure 6.2: A family tree showing inheritance of an autosomal dominant disease. Individuals III,4 and III,5 asked to be evaluated for their genetic risk to develop the disease

In the reported example, the father of individuals III,4 and III,5 is affected. Therefore he must carry the defective allele. The probability of having received such allele from the father will be 0,5 (50%) for each of the two sibs.

In case of traits with reduced penetrance, computation must be corrected accordingly. For instance, if gene determining the above disease would be 70% penetrant, the probability of developing a *manifested* disease will be for each proband (70%)x(50%) = 35% (i.e. 65% probability of being healthy through all his/her life).

However, usually the risk of developing the disease is more precisely calculated by Bayesian logic.

Let's consider the case of an apparently healthy individual, aged 55, whose mother developed at the age of 50 a genetic disease inherited as a mendelian autosomal dominant trait. The manifestation of this disease is known to occur in the adult age, between the ages of 40 and 60.

The probability of having inherited the defective gene is called "prior" probability, since it derives from the knowledge of the family history.

In this case, the prior probability of having inherited the disease will be 0.5 (50%). Let's also suppose that 90% (0.9) of cases show typical symptoms before the age of 55. Therefore, the probability of not showing symptoms at the age of 55, albeit having inherited the defective allele, will be 0.10 (1-0.9). This probability is called "conditional probability". Conditional probability of manifesting no symptoms being not affected will be obviously 1. By multiplication of prior probability by conditional probability, a "joint probability" is obtained. Two joint probabilities must be computed, one under the hypothesis that the proband inherited the defective allele ("affected"), the other under the hypothesis that he inherited the normal allele from his mother ("unaffected").

Once joints probabilities are computed, "posterior" (final) probability is obtained as the ratio between joint probability of having inherited the defective allele and the sum of the two joint probabilities (of having inherited and of not having inherited the defective allele, respectively).

In the case considered by the example, the situation will be the following:

PROBABILITY	"AFFECTED"	"UNAFFECTED"
Prior (genetic)	0.5	0.5
Conditional	0.1	1
Joint	0.05	0.5
Posterior	0.09	

Therefore, the proband risk is below 10%.

Often, additional information is available, based on clinical phenotype, on tests results, or, more simply, on the individual' offspring or kindred. From each available information a conditional probability may be calculated for each of the two alternative hypotheses (having or not having inherited the disease-allele).

Let's consider the following case:

The proband's father died of acute coronary atherosclerotic disease (CAD). At the time of consultation the proband is 45 years old and he shows a cholesterol positive test (above 240 mg/dl). Let's assume that sensitivity of the cholesterol test is 0.75 and specificity is 0.9. Let's assume also that the proband was found to carry the ACE D/D genotype (0.45 sensitivity and 0.72 specificity, according to data reported by Keavney on a very large sample of cases and controls).

In this case, prior probability cannot be calculated from the Mendel's rules, being the disease multifactorial. However, empiric data are available, telling that genetic risk of developing coronary CAD for a person showing a positive family history for the disease is about 1/5 (0.2).

We may take this value as our best estimate of prior probability of having inherited the "at-risk" genotype.

Conditional probability of developing CAD, associated with a positive (>240 mg/dl) cholesterol test result corresponds to sensitivity of the test (0.75), while conditional probability of not developing CAD will be (1- 0.9), i.e. (1- specificity).

The same reasoning is applied to the result of genetic test.

Then, situation is the following:

PROBABILITY	"AFFECTED"	"UNAFFECTED"
Prior (genetic)	0.2	0.8
Conditional 1 (Chol)	0.75	0.1
Conditional 2 (marker)	0.45	0.28
Joint	0.0675	0.0224
Posterior	0.75	

In this case, the proband has a very high probability (75%) of developing CAD.

It is interesting to note that prior probability plus information on cholesterol level contribute to 86% of the final risk value.

It should be also noted that in the above example, carrying the ACE DD genotype would increase the risk from 0.65 to 0.75.

If a genetic test would have been available, showing the same sensitivity and specificity as the cholesterol test, in the same situation (positive family history, plus positive cholesterol test, plus positive genetic test), the risk would have been 0.93!

Bayesan logic may be applied to any problem of genetic risk assessment, provided sufficient information is available to compute conditional probabilities. It should be noted that the more numerous *independent* conditional probabilities could be evaluated, the more precise would be the final risk estimate.

<u>Detection of a pathogenic mutation in a healthy subject</u> poses serious problems about precise evaluation of his risk of developing the disease. Data about age of manifestation of the disease, age-related penetrance, variability in clinical severity and therapeutical perspectives should be considered with great attention. Moreover, genetic counselling is useful in most cases.

6.5 Genetic tests: some ethical and legal aspects

Genetic tests always involve ethical and legal aspects, since information on DNA is, by definition, the most private information, from which additional information may be obtained about biological descent.

A report on genetics and privacy was recently produced by California HealthCare Foundation (Hustead, 2002)

Before a blood sample is taken for DNA analysis, a written and explicit consent should be obtained from the involved person. In the signed form, clear statements should be included, about exclusive usage of the DNA sample for purposes indicated in the form, confidentiality of information, and protection of individual data stored in databases. If the DNA sample would be stored in a DNA bank, an additional written consent should be obtained, in which conditions of banking (property of the sample, conditions for futher analysis, possibility of withdrawing the sample, etc) should be clearly stated.

Not always direct DNA "diagnosis" (i.e. detection of causative mutations in the considered gene) is possible. The disease gene could be still unknown, in spite of having been mapped to a specific chromosomal region; in other cases its very large size, wide heterogeneity of its mutations or failure of preliminary mutation screening may justify an "indirect" approach. In such instances, and when additional cases are present in the family, not only proband's DNA, but DNA samples of as many as possible of his/her relatives should be collected and analyzed, in order to perform linkage analysis or haplotype study.

Blood sampling for DNA analysis may be *prescribed* for diagnostic purposes only to persons who are otherwise suspected to be affected with a disease. Therefore, this applies only to other affected members in the family. On the contrary, DNA tests cannot be prescribed to healthy relatives of a proband; blood samples from them may be obtained only on voluntary basis.

People are very concerned about possible malpractice in handling DNA data; actually, familiar data are very sensitive, because they provide the most direct evidence of biological parenthood. Moreover, DNA data might be possibly used against an unaware person, for discrimination or even in legal cases. Several family members could refuse to participate in the study, for the above reasons or, more simply because they fear to be detected positive for a pathogenic mutation. Finally, even contacting family members in order to ask their collaboration to a genetic investigation may be felt as an undue invasion of the privacy. Therefore, several difficulties are often encountered in genetic studies concerning families.

The problem may be approached by a multi-step process:

1) Explanation to proband that his problem (risk assessment) could not be solved, unless the collaboration of his relatives could be obtained; he should contact his relatives and explain them the conditions of their possible collaboration;

2) Clear definition of the conditions of collaboration, in a written informed consent form specimen, to be handed by the proband to each relative; this form includes statements about exclusive usage of the DNA sample for purposes indicated in the form, on strict privacy and confidentiality of information on genetic status, on protection of data stored in databases and on storing or disposal of individual DNA samples. One sentence should clarify whether or not the involved person wishes to be informed about results of the analyses on his/her DNA. In any case, no one family member could have access to information regarding his/her relatives, except his/her infant sibs.

3) Contact by each relative who accepted in principle to collaborate, for further information about participation in the study.

4) Signature of the informed consent(s) and blood sampling.

5) Communication of results of DNA analyses to those who explicitly asked for it.

In general, infant or teenagers are not included in family studies, first of all because in several diseases manifestation of clinical phenotype occurs in the adult age, secondly because of ethical and legal problems.

Blood sampling in infants or teenagers require authorization from both parents or, in absence of them, from the legal tutor. It may be difficult to obtain the authorization from both parents, especially if they are divorced.

Although parents may be strongly emotionally involved in facts concerning their sibs, their right to know the genotype of their children is restricted to diseases manifested in childhood or in early adult age, i.e. during the period of time in which parents are legally responsible for their sibs. This restriction is justified by the assumption that life of a child would be different in presence or absence of genetic information about a severe disease which he could develop in the adult age. For instance, parents might plan a different investment for a child in which an "affected" genotype was detected, in respect to a child with a "normal" genotype. Such a discrimination is particularly unjust, since the sib showing a normal genotype for the gene investigated might in reality carry a defect in a different, but univestigated gene. Moreover, present perspectives of possible treatment or therapy for a person affected with a given genetic disease, might change in the near future, due to progress of molecular Medicine.

To patients, genetic test are not equivalent to biochemical tests, in spite they are "laboratory tests". A biochemical alteration revealed by a laboratory test, even the presence of a cancer marker, is interpreted as evidence of an adverse circumstance, which could be hopefully corrected. On the contrary, the result of a genetic test is felt as the revelation of an unalterable situation. For this reason, communication of results of genetic tests should be better part of a process of genetic counselling, rather than of clinical diagnosis.

Terms: *affected genotype* and *disease gene* should be avoided when explaining results of genetic tests to a patient; *at-risk genetic makeup* and *gene involved in the disease* should be used instead (in fact, this latter expression is more correct than *disease gene*, if we consider the role of genetic background and of environmental factors in producing a clinical phenotype).

6.6 Genetics and genomics applied to drug therapy: pharmacogenetics and pharmacogenomics

Pharmacogenetics is the study of the genetic component of individual response to drugs. Parmacogenomics is a novel discipline, dealing with the application of pharmacogenetics and genomic concepts to drug discovery and drug clinical development.

Pharmacogenetics started as a discipline in the mid-1950's, when pseudocholinesterase variation was found to cause suxamethonium sensitivity and anomalies in erytrhrocyte glutathione metabolism were reported in primaquine sensitivity. Since then, several genetic variations were described, which cause altered response to specific drugs.

When a cohort of patients is treated with a given drug, the observed variability in the individual response may be due to genetic heterogeneity, but, more probably, to inter-individual variation in pharmacokinetics (Nakagawa, 2000)

Drug uptake, transport, biotransformation and excretion, depend on specific proteins acting as enzymes, binding factors or carriers. Since such proteins may show genetic variants, variability in pharmacokinetics among patients must be always expected.

On the other hand, it is known that administration of a specific drug may produce disease in carriers of genetic variants of specific genes; these variants are said "conditionally pathogenic", since no disease would be manifested in absence of the specific drug treatment. Some examples of this situation are reported in Tab. 6.2.

Table 6.2: Some "classical" pharmacogenetic conditions and drugs producing the abnormal response (I: mode of inheritance; AD: autosomal dominant; AR: autosomal recessive; XD: X-linked dominant; XR, X-linked recessive)

Condition	I	Drug
Acatalasia	AR	Hydrogen peroxide
Acetophenetidin-induced methemoglobinemia	AR	Acetophenetidin
Drug-sensitives hemoglobins (Hb-Zurich; Hb-H)	AD	Sulfonamides
Dyphenylhydantoin toxicity	AD	Dyphenylhydantoin
Dyphenylhydantoin toxicity	XD	Dyphenylhydantoin
G6PD deficiency/drug-induced hemolytic anemia	XD	Many drugs
Glaucoma induced by steroids	AR	Corticosteroids
Malignant hyperthermia	AD	Halothane
Neurotoxicity (slow inactivation of isoniazide)	AR	Isoniazide
Suxamethonium sensitivity	AR	Suxamethonium
Warfarin resistance	AR	Warfarin

Over 60 pharmacogenetic differences were reported so far (Nebert, 1999). If we except cases of pharmacogenetic diseases, where the presence of genetic variant may be inferred from phenotype, genetic variability in the response to drugs is usually obscured by many intrinsic and environmental factors, among which individual age, sex, biorythms, disease and interaction of the considered molecule with other drugs or with endogenous or exogenous compounds (Bozler, 1978). Therefore, response to a given drug must be considered a phenotype due to multifactorial determination.

It has been estimated that poor response to treatment with expensive drugs and adverse drug effects cost about 100 billion US$ and 100,000 deaths per year, in the US. Therefore, individual genotyping predicting the risk of a severely adverse drug effect or the failure of a given therapy is presently viewed as a very important possible application of DNA tests. However, due to multifactorial determination of response to drugs, this method is expected to be really beneficial only in a minority of patients (Ingelman-Sundberg, 2001).

6.7 Pharmacogenetics in Cardiology

Some drugs currently used in clinical practice may produce adverse effects in individuals carrying a conditionally pathogenic variant. For instance, administration of acetyl-salicilic acid or of trinitrotoluene to carriers of Glucose-6-phosphate deficiency may be unsafe.

On the other hand, known antiarrythmic drugs may induce or worsen arrhythmias. It may be supposed that individual variation in drug clearance could increase plasma concentration of the administered drug, thus potentially triggering adverse effects. Also variations in drug metabolism in liver, due to genetic or environmental factors, may reduce drug clearance, making a supposedly well-tolerated dose toxic (Woosley, 1987).

Actually, a number of drugs belonging to different therapeutic classes (antiarrhythmic, antibiotic, antifungal, antihistamine, antipsychotic, prokinetic drugs, etc) share in common the property of inducing a prolongation of cardiac re-polarization, thus exposing patients to risk of torsade de pointes, sincope and sudden death. This adverse effect seems to occur in a subset of susceptible patients, which show an increased risk of arrhythmias upon exposure to any of such drugs. It was suspected that susceptible patients could carry a silent (non pathogenic, in absence of treatment) mutation in one of the genes involved in the determination of long-QT syndrome (Escande, 2000). On the other hand, different non-antiarrhythmic drugs at risk of inducing torsade de pointes were found to be primarily metabolized by cytochrome P450 isozymes 34A and 2D6 and it was hypothesized that risk of developing torsade de pointes is due to variants of such proteins (Bauman, 2001).

The occurrence of a lupus-like syndrome in a significant number of patients treated with procainamide has limited the clinical use of this antiarrhythmic drug. Inter-individual variability in procainamide metabolism has been reported, possibly involving CYP2D6, the major cytochrome P450 isozyme involved in the formation of N-hydroxyprocainamide, which is believed to be linked to the induction of the lupus-like syndrome (Lessard, 1999). Therefore, CYP2D6 seems to play a very important role in determining differences in response to treatment with several drugs currently used in cardiological clinical practice.

Acetyl-salicilic acid is widely used to reduce the risk of platelet aggregation, but this treatment is not equally effective in all patients. It has been suggested that carriers of an infrequent variant of the gene P1A2, encoding a platelet glycoprotein, could be more responsive to aspirin treatment than others (Goldschmidt-Clermont, 1999).

Although pharmacogenetics is still almost at its beginning, the number of scientific publications on this subject, dealing with treatment of cardiovascular disorders doubled in the last three years. Presently, attention is mostly focused on detecting and analyzing genes involved in the response to

ACE-inhibitors, beta-adrenoreceptor antagonists, angiotensin receptor antagonists, sprironolactone, vasopeptidase inhibitors and endothelin receptor antagonists.

A current approach is to type each patient for a series of genetic variations (mostly SNPs) in genes presumably relevant to the phenotype (e.g. effective response or, conversely, uneffective response) and then check whether a particular type of response could be associated to a given pattern of variations.

This approach recalls the strategy used to detect genes involved in multifactorial disorders (Chapter 3, Section 3.4) and shares with it all pros and cons.

I would like to conclude this Section with the citation of a prudent, authoritative and thoughtful sentence: "not all drug responses are determined by inheritance and not all genetically determined responses will be easy to measure" (Wilkins, 2000).

6.8 Pharmacogenomics and beyond

In pharmacogenomics, understanding individual variability in response to treatment with a given drug is approached by means of expression studies simultaneously performed on a large number of genes, or by other sophisticated genomic methods.

In principle, pharmacogenomics, being a massive investigation on genome, should be free from selection biases; moreover being a high-throughput approach, it should provide a sufficiently large number of data for further and successful analysis.

The aim of current studies in this field is to describe genomic profiles of drug sensitivities. While this is a very difficult task in humans, both because of costs and ethical problems, it may be feasible in other experimental systems. For instance, a set of heterozygous yeast strains carrying deletions in genes encoding known drug targets were constructed. Each heterozygous strain was tested by growth in the presence of sublethal concentration of the drug directly targeting the protein encoded by the locus heterozygous for the deletion. Experiments conducted on different strains showed that, if a heterozygous yeast strain exhibits increased sensitivity to a given drug, manifested by reduced fitness, then the heterozygous gene may encode the drug target. Thus, drug-sensitivity profiling of many different strains enables to detect drug-sensitive loci. In this experimental system no *a priori* knowledge of the target is required; only those targets which affect the fitness of yeast strain will be identified (Giaver, 1999).

The advancement of comparative genomics provides the opportunity of transferring knowledge acquired on a relatively simple experimental system, like yeast, to different and more complex systems, like invertebrates or mammals.

As we have seen in Chapter 2, Section 2.3, once genes and proteins would be identified, next step will be identification of their interactions in the metabolic network. Correlation of gene expression data and protein-protein interaction data will enable to link functional genomics to metabolic phenotyping. This approach will be particularly helpful in understanding clinical pharmacology and pharmacogenetics.

On the other hand, this basic knowledge should help in identifying novel drug targets. It is assumed that only a small fractions of human genes might code for drug target proteins: possibly proteins involved in disease pathway are not so many and probably only some of them would be suitable to bind a small molecule, devised for therapeutic purposes.

The development of robust, automated mass spectrometry technology, coupled with availability of complete genome sequences and with the development of tools for comparing mass spectrometry data to sequence data will give new impulse to protein profiling.

Genomics, proteomics and informatics are creating novel opportunities for investigation on molecular pathogenesis of several human diseases, with particular reference to identification of prognostic markers, drug development and response to therapy.

6.9 Gene-based therapeutics

Identification and cloning of genes, recombinant DNA technology (i.e. inserting a selected DNA sequence in a foreign DNA) and methods of cell manipulation opened the way to gene transfer from one organism to another. In Chapter 4 (Section 4.5) we have seen how this technology may be used to create transgenic animals.

The same principles were applied to develop novel therapies for human diseases, based on gene transfer. Therapeutic strategies based on gene transfer arc listed in Tab. 6.3.

Table 6.3: Diffcrent therapeutical strategies, bascd on gene transfer.

AIM	STRATEGY
Restore normal function in genetically defective cells	Introduction of extra copies of a given gene in order to increase concentration of corresponding protein to a level at which normal phenotype is restored
Targeted cell killing	Introduction of a gene, which product is toxic or letal for the targeted cell
Correction of a disease-causing mutation	Replacement of defective copy of a gene by a normal copy, by homologous recombination

The general aim is to treat a diseasc by delivering foreign genetic material to target cells, where the novel genetic information could be released. For instance, normal copies of a given gene could be delivered to defective cells of a person affected with a genetic disease. Normal genes, once inside target cells, would produce normal proteins and could remediate the defect.

Conversely, genes producing a toxic product or promoting cell death might be transferred to cancer cells and could hopefully kill them. Alternatively, foreign genes might be transferred, which produce a pro-drug, thus conferring to target cells high sensitivity to a specific drug.

Targeted mutation correction, i.e. replacement of a defective gene copy by a normal one, which is currently achieved in mice, is still encountering in humans many practical difficulties and some ethical objections.

Genes can be trasferred to target cells by a "vector". Viral vectors (usually engineered adenoviruses) will carry the foreign gene as an "insert" in their DNA, while non viral vectors (usually liposomes, i.e. vesicles made by synthetic lipid bilayers) carry DNA in form of DNA-lipid complexes.

Viral vectors show high efficiency of gene transfer, but they may elicit immune response in the infected organism, whereas non viral vectors are safe from this point of view, but they are much less efficient in transfection.

Gene delivery to target cells may be achieved *in vivo*, by administation of vectors to the patient to be treated, by direct injection in the tissue or by infusion. In some cases, an *ex-vivo* delivery is possible: cells obtained from the patient are cultured in vitro, transfected and then returned to the patient.

This procedure recently attracted novel interest, after exciting progresses were made in the field of stem cells transplantation. Stem cells could be genetically modified in vitro and then transplanted into the target tissue.

The idea of applying gene therapy to myocardial diseases dates back to the early 90's. In fact, heart appears particularly suitable for application of gene therapy, being a relatively small organ, highly vascularized and accessible by catheters. Different ways of delivery were tested in dogs: direct myocardial injection, coronary artery perfusion and intrapericardial injection. As expected, coronary artery perfusion appeared the less harmful method, though producing a sparse expression of the transgene carried by an adenoviral vector. Direct myocardial injection of the vector produced significant expression of the transgene, but concentrated around the injection site and was accompanied by local inflammatory response. Intrapericardial cavity injection of the vector produced detectable expression of the transgene in the inner surface of the pericardium, epicardial surface of the heart and partially in the myocardium underneath (Li, 2002). In humans, gene transfer to the arrested heart during cardiopulmonary bypass may represent another alternative (Jones, 2002). Different methods of delivery may meet different therapeutic aims, e.g. treating the epicardium, a localized myocardial alteration or the entire myocardium.

Studies conducted on laboratory animals produced encouraging results. There is evidence that myocardial gene therapy in rats improves cardiac performance in heart failure and suceeds in prolonging life of treated animals (del Monte, 2001). On the other hand, intracoronary administration of replication-defective adenoviruses carrying a human fibroblast growth factor (FGF) gene appeared to be safe and effective in a double-blind randomized trial in patients with stable angina pectoris (Grines, 2002).

Gene therapy of some cardiovascular diseases in humans is a realistic perspective in the near future. Optimistic views were expressed also on possible development of gene therapy of arrhythmic disorders (Carmeliet, 2001).

Before gene therapy could become a tool in clinical cardiology, several important problems should be solved: selection of a suitable, safe and efficient vector; selection of the most suitable, safe and efficient way of administration of vector; efficient transfer of transgenes to cardiomyocytes after administration of vector; stability and activity of transgenes within target cells, safety of repeated administration of vectors to patients and, last but not least, therapeutic efficacy of the adopted protocols.

A different kind of therapeutics is based on targeted inhibition of gene expression. Such inibition may be achieved at DNA, RNA or protein level.

It is possible to design oligonucleotides which could form triple-helix structures in combination with specific segments of double-helix DNA. If the designed oligonucleotide is specific for the promoter region of a given gene, formation of triple-helix would impede transcription. TFO (Triplex-Forming Oligonucleotides) are a promising class of potential "genetic" therapeutics.

Messenger RNA is single-stranded. If a mRNA meets its "antisense" (i.e. its complementary sequence), binding would inhibit translation. In some cases mRNA bound to its antisense is quickly degraded within the cell.

It is interesting to note that natural antisense RNAs probably plays a physiological role in the regulation of several mammalian genes, including Troponin I and Myosin heavy chain in the human myocardium (Luther, 2001; Podlowski, 2002).

It is now possible to produce "antisense genes", i.e. genes whose transcripts are antisense of given mRNAs. Transfer of an antisense gene to a target cell will ensure adequate intracellular concentration of the antisense RNA, thus producing selective inhibition of translation of a given mRNA.

Synthetic antisense Oligo-DeoxyriboNucleotides (ODNs) are in general preferred, because of their chemical stability. Resistance to cellular nucleases may be enhanced by chemical modification of theODN molecule ends.

ODNs were successfully used in different instances. In an experiment in vitro on myocardiocytes from failing human hearts, infection with adenoviruses encoding the antisense of Phospholamban (PL) gene succeeded in ablating PL function and in restoring the normal frequency response in myocardiocytes, thus demonstrating that targeting phospholamban may provide therapeutic benefits in heart failure (del Monte, 2002).

Antisense therapy was proposed to reduce neointima formation in restenosis (Kipshidze, 2002), to decrease matrix protein production and secretion (Weiss, 2002) or even to control hypertension (Sellers, 2001).

A different way of inhibiting expression of a specific gene may be achieved by transfer of an artificial gene encoding a "ribozyme" , i.e. a RNA molecule including a short sequence ("hammerhead") showing catalytic properties. Once base-pairing is established between ribozyme sequence and the sequence of target mRNA, the catalytic part of the ribozyme promotes cleavage with subsequent inactivation of mRNA and, therefore, ablation of gene expression.

Finally, inhibition at protein level may be achieved by aid of the so-called "intrabodies", i.e. intracellular antibodies. It is possible to design artificial genes encoding such kind of proteins, which can bind and inactivate specific proteins within the cell.

List in Tab. 6.4 is not exhaustive, but it may give a preliminary information on a novel generation of therapeutics. Some of them (TFOs, ODNs) may be considered real drugs, since they directly interfere in a biochemical process. On the contrary, transferred genes are peculiar drugs, since their therapeutical effects are due to proteins encoded by them, but produced by cells in which DNAs were transferred.

Table 6.4: Different types of genetic therapeutics and their effects.

METHOD	EFFECT
Gene transfer	Adds normal copies of a given gene
Gene transfer	Adds gene, encoding toxin
Gene transfer	Adds gene, encoding pro-drug
Gene transfer	Adds gene, encoding antisense
Gene transfer	Adds gene, encoding ribozyme
Gene transfer	Adds gene, encoding intrabodies
TFO	Binds to a specific promoter
ODN	Binds to a specific mRNA
Ribozyme	Binds to a specific mRNA
Intrabody	Binds to a specific protein

In summary, gene transfer of additional copies of a given gene or of an artificial gene capable of permanent expression will help in treating diseases due to deficit of a given gene product. On the contrary, administration of TFOs, ODNs, or transfer of a gene encoding an antisense RNA or a ribozyme, may succeed in counteracting unwanted hyperexpression of a given gene. Gene transfer of genes encoding toxins or pro-drugs can be helpful in situations in which hyperproliferation of cells should be controlled.

Transient expression of transgenes, which is considered a big limitation when attempting to cure severe Mendelian disorders, is an advantage when dealing with disorders due to temporary de-regulation of some genes. In this case, limitation in time of transgene expression is desired, in order to avoid persistency of its effects, once clinical situation would be restored to normal.

Present investigations on genomic expression profiles of myocardial tissue in health and disease will likely lead to identification of abnormally upregulated genes in specific cardiac diseases, thus paving the way for clinical application of genetic therapeutics. Even Mendelian disorders could possibly benefit from these studies, since restoring the normal pattern of genomic expression, altered by a genetically determined metabolic defect, should reduce the severity of clinical symptoms.

SUMMARY Development of molecular genetics and genomics will soon have a strong impact on medical practice. Molecular genetic investigations are already part of diagnostic procedure in several cardiomyopathies and arrhythmogenic disorders. In these cases, identification of the involved gene and of the causative mutation may help in defining prognosis and possibly in selection of a proper treatment. DNA testing may be used as well for identifying individuals at risk to develop a given disease (pre-symptomatic testing). Ethical and legal aspects of this procedure must be carefully considered. Great interest was raised by the possibility of predictive DNA testing for cardiovascular disorders. Such tests are still in an early phase of development. Their sensitivity, specificity, positive and negative predictive values, clinical validity and clinical utility must be evaluated before they could be introduced in the clinical practice. A different field of research, fuelled by genomics and molecular genetics, is pharmacogenetics, i.e. the study of genetic basis of individual response to drugs.   ->

Several drugs induce a prolongation of cardiac re-polarization in a subset of susceptible patients. The development of genetic tests for detecting such susceptibility or other situation of differential response to given drugs would be highly beneficial.

Identification of human genes, coupled with methods of gene manipulation and gene transfer, opened the way to gene-based therapeutics, aiming at restoring normal function in genetically defective cells, at correcting disease-causing mutations, or even at killing specific cells. Viral and non-viral vectors for delivering foreign DNA to cells were developed in the last decade; moreover, novel strategies were devised, based on inhibition of expression of selected genes, by using antisense or triplex-forming oligonucleotides. Heart is particularly suitable for the application of gene-based therapeutics. Preliminary experiments and double-blind trials produced encouraging results.

Conclusion

For about 50 years, research in biochemistry, cell biology and physiology considerably increased our understanding about mechanisms underlying heart function in health and disease. As a consequence, rational therapeutical strategies were devised, which have significantly improved the management of cardiac diseases.

In the last decade, Molecular Genetics made relevant progresses in detecting genes involved in Mendelian cardiomyopathies and inherited arrhythmogenic diseases, thus enabling to attempt genetic dissection of pathogenesis in heart diseases.

Genomic Medicine is now bringing novel impulse to this line of research. The hypothesis of "final common pathways" leading to manifestation of given clinical phenotypes is being now implemented by expression data concerning specific genes involved in different steps of given pathways

Disease is now viewed as an alteration of genomic expression profile in a given tissue, rather than as consequence of a single, isolated defect. Therefore, our understanding is shifting from the original deterministic model toward a very complex network model.

Mastering this complexity would be impossible without the help of computers. In the course of the Human Genome race, bioinformatics gained experience and credit and, at the end, it was the real winner of the race. Presently, bioinformatics is tackling the difficult problem of putting together an enormous amount of data, to reconstruct a realistic representation of biological phenomena, in a sort of reverse engineering. The so-called "In-silico Biology" is attempting not only to interpret changes in genomic expression using molecular interaction networks, but also to simulate very complex biochemical interactions at intracellular and inter-cellular level. An interesting example of such approach is the so-called E-CELL project, at the website http://www.bioinformatics.org/e-cell/.

Recent advancements in mathematical biology and modelling created new opportunities for the construction of computational frameworks enabling to build up models suitable for simulations. The perspective that mathematical models of a simplified cell or of a simple multicellular organism could be soon available is not unrealistic. Such models might be profitably used also for understanding pathogenesis or the effects of specific drugs.

Researches on computational models of failing myocyte (Winslow, 2001) and of heart performance (Kohl, 1999) are now in progress. Integrative modelling of cardiac function and parallel computing for the numerical solution of large systems of equations, produced very interesting and encouraging results (Winslow, 2001). The making of a virtual heart is ahead, on which heart failure could be simulated and the effect of novel drugs could be tested (Kohl, 2001).

We may envisage that data obtained from genomic, proteomic and metabolomic research would progressively ameliorate the predictive power of such models, thus opening a new era of cardiological research and providing novel perpectives to therapy.

REFERENCES

Adams M.D. et al. Sequence identification of 2,375 human brain genes. Nature 355: 632-634, 1992

Adams M.D. et al. Rapid cDNA sequencing (expressed sequence tags) from a directionally cloned human infant brain cDNA library. Nature Genetics 4: 373-380, 1993

Alings M. et al. Brugada syndrome. Clinical data and suggested pathophysiological mechanism. Circulation 99: 666-673, 1999

Allayee H. et al. Genome scan for blood pressure in Dutch dyslipidemic families reveals linkage to a locus on chromosome 4p. Hypertension 38: 773-778, 2001

Andreotti F. et al. Inflammatory gene polymorphisms and ischaemic heart disease: review of population association studies. Heart 87: 107-112, 2002

Antonarakis S.A. Recommendations for a nomenclature system for human gene mutations. Hum. Mutat. 11: 1-3, 1988

Arca M. et al. Autosomal recessive hypercholesterolaemia in Sardinia, Italy, and mutations in ARH: a clinical and molecular genetic analysis. Lancet 359: 841-847, 2002

Arngrimsson R. et al. A genome-wide scan reveals a maternal susceptibility locus for pre-ecclampsia on chromosome 2p13. Hum.Molec.Gen. 8: 1799-1805, 1999

Aronow B.J. et al. Divergent transcriptional responses to independent genetic causes of cardiac hypertrophy. Physiol.Genomics 1: 19-28, 2001

Atwood L.D. et al. Genome-wide linkage analysis of blood pressure in Mexican Americans. Genet.Epidem. 20: 373-382, 2001

Barrans J.D. et al. Construction of a human cardiovascular cDNA microarray: portrait of the failing heart. Biochem. Biophys. Res. Commun. 280: 964-969, 2001

Bauman J.L. The role of pharmacokinetics, drug interactions and pharmacogenetics in the acquired long-QT syndrome. Eur.Heart J. Suppl. 3: K93-K100, 2001

Benetos A. et al. Influence of Angiotensin-II type 1 receptor gene polymorphism on aortic stiffness in never-treated hypertensive patients. Hypertension 26: 44-47, 1995

Bonnardeaux A. et al. The Angiotensin II type 1 receptor gene polymorphism in human essential hypertension. Hypertension 24:63-69, 1994

Bortoluzzi S. et al. A computational reconstruction of the adult human heart transcriptional profile. J.Mol.Cell.Cardiol. 32: 1931-1938, 2000

Bozler G. Human pharmacokinetics. In: "Human Genetic Variation in response to Medical and Environmental Agents: Pharmacogenetics and Ecogenetics. Hum.genet., Suppl. 1: 13-17, 1978

Brand E. et al. Evaluation of the angiotensin locus in human hypertension: an European study. Hypertension 31: 725-729, 1998

Bray M.S. et al. The role of beta-2 adrenergic receptor variation in human hypertension. Curr. Hypertens. Rep. 2: 39-43, 2000

Broeckel U. et al. A comprehensive linkage analysis for myocardial infarction and its related risk factors. Nature Genet. 30: 210-214, 2002

Cambien F. et al. Deletion polymorphism in the gene for angiotensin-converting enzyme is a potent risk factor for myocardial infarction., Nature 359: 641-644, 1992

Carmeliet E. et al. New approaches to antiarrhythmic therapy: emerging therapeutical applications of the cell biology of cardiac arrhythmias. Cardiovasc. Res. 52: 345-360, 2001

Chin A.J. Congenital heart disease. In: Principles of Molecular Medicine. J.L. Jameson et al. Eds. Humana Press Inc. Totowa, NJ, 1998 pp 117-125

Cooke R.A. et al. Noonan's cardiomyopathy: a non-hypertrophic variant. Brit.Heart J. 71:561-565, 1994

Coon H. et al. Genome-wide linkage analysis of hypertension Genetic epidemiology Network (HyperGEN) blood Pressure study. Arter. Thromb.Vasc. Biol. 21: 1969-1976, 2001

Croft S.A. et al. Novel platelet membrane glycoprotein VI polymorphism is a risk factor for myocardial infarction. Circulation 104: 1459-1463, 2001

Cvetkovic B. & Sigmund C.D. Understanding hypertension through genetic manipulation in mice. Kidn.Internat. 57: 863-874, 2000

Danieli G.A. & Rampazzo A. Genetics of Arrhythmogenic Right Ventricular Cardiomyopathy. Curr. Opin. Cardiol. 17 : 218-221, 2002

Davisson R.L. et al. Discovery of a sponteneous genetic mouse model of preecclampsia. Hypertension 39: 337-342, 2002

del Monte F. et al. Improvement in survival and cardiac metabolism after gene transfer of sarcoplasmic reticulum Ca++ATPase in a rat model of heart failure. Circulation 104: 1424-1429, 2001

del Monte F. et al. Targeting phospholamban by gene transfer in human heart failure. Circulation 105: 904-907, 2002

Doris P.A. Hypertension genetics, single nucleotide polymorphisms and the common disease: common variant hypothesis Hypertension 39: 323-331, 2002

Dumaine R. & Antzelevitch C. Molecular mechanisms underlying the long QT syndrome. Curr. Opin. Cardiol. 17: 36-42, 2002

Escande D. Pharmacogenetics of cardiac K+ channels. Eur. J. Pharmacol. 410: 281-287, 2000

Feld S. & Caspi A. Familial cardiomyopathy with variable hypertrophic and restrictive features and common HLA haplotype. Israel J.Med.Sci. 28: 277-280, 1992

Fernandez-Arcas N. et al. Both alleles of the M235T of the angiotensinogen gene can be a risk factor for myocardial infarction. Clin. Genet. 60: 52-57, 2001

Ferrandi M. et al. Evidence for an interaction between Adducin and Na+K+ ATPase: relation to genetic hypertension. Lancet 349: 1353-1357, 1997

Fitzpatrick A.P. et al. Familial restrictive cardiomyopathy with atrioventricular block and skeletal myopathy. Brit. Heart. J. 63: 114-118, 1990

Fontaine G. et al. Arrhythmogenic right ventricular dysplasia. Annu.Rev. Med. 50: 17-35, 1999

Francke S. et al. A genome-wide scan for coronary heart disease suggests in Indo-Mauritians a susceptibility locus on chromosome 16p13 and replicates linkage with the metabolic syndrome on 3q27. Hum.Molec.Genet. 10: 2751-2765, 2001

Franco D, et al. The transcriptional building blocks of the heart. In "Cardiovascular specific gene expression" P.A. Doevendans, R.S. Reneman and M. van Bilsen Eds., Kluwer Academic Publishers, Dordrecht, The Netherlands, 1999, pp 7-16

Franz W.M et al. Cardiomyopathies: from genetics to the prospect of treatment. The Lancet 358: 1627-1637, 2001

Friddle C.J. et al. Expression profiling reveals distinct sets of genes altered during induction an regression of cardiac hypertrophy. Proc. Natl. Acad.Sci. US 97: 6754-6750, 2000

Geller D.S. et al. Activating mineralocorticoid receptor mutation in hypertension exacerbated by pregnancy. Science 289: 119-123, 2000

Giaver G. et al. Genomic profiling of drug sensitivities via induced haploinsufficiency. Nature Genet. 21: 278-283, 1999

Girelli D. et al. Polymorphisms in the Factor VII gene and the risk of myocardial infarction in patients with coronary artery disease. New Engl.J.Med. 343: 774-780, 2000

Goldschmidt-Clermont P.J. et al. Platelet P1A2 polymorphism and thromboembolic events: from inherited risk to pharmacogenetics. J. Thromb. Thrombol. 8: 89-103, 1999

Grines C.L. et al. Angiogenic GENe Therapy (AGENT) trial in patients with stable angina pectoris. Circulation 105: 1291-1297, 2002

Gudnason V. et al. Common founder mutation in the LDL-receptor gene causing familial hypercholesterolemia in the Icelandic population. Hum.Mutat. 10: 36-44, 1997

Harrap S.B. et al. Blood pressure QTLs identified by genome-wide linkage analysis and dependence on associated phenotypes. Physiol. Genomics 8: 99-105, 2002

Hetet G. et al. Association studies between haemochromatosis gene mutations and the risk of cardiovascular diseases. Eur. J. Clin. Invest. 31: 382-388, 2001

Hirschhorn J.N. et al. A comprehensive review of genetic association studies. Genet.in Med. 4: 45-61, 2002

Ho C.Y. et al. Homozygous mutation in Cardiac Troponin T. Implications for hypertrophic cardiomyopathy. Circulation 102: 1950, 2000

Hokanson J.E. et al. Lipoprotein lipase gene variants and risk of coronary disease: a quantitative analysis of population-based studies. Int. J. Clin. Lab.Res. 27: 24-34, 1997

Hsueh W.C. et al. QTL influencing bood pressure maps to the region PPH1 on chromosome 2q31-34 in Old Order Amish. Circulation 101: 2810-2816, 2000

Hustead J.L. et al. Genetics and Privacy: a patchwork of protections. California HeathCare Foundation, 2002

Hwang D.M. et al. A genome-based resource for molecular cardiovascular medicine: toward a compendium of cardiovascular genes. Circulation 96: 4146-4203, 1997

Hwang D.M. et al. Identification of differentially expressed genes in cardiac hypertrophy by analysis of expressed sequence tags. Genomics 66: 1-4, 2000

Ingelman-Sundberg M. Pharmacogenetics: an opportunity for a safer and more efficient pharmacotherapy. J.Internal Med. 250: 186-200, 2001

Inoue I. et al. A nucleotide substitution in the promoter of human angiotensinogen is associated with essential hypertension and affects basal transcription in vitro. J.Clin. Invest. 99: 1786-1797, 1999

Ishiwata S. et al. Restrictive cardiomyopathy with complete atrioventricular block and distal myopathy with rimmed vacuoles. Jpn. Circ. J. 57: 928-933, 1993

Jeunemaitre X. et al. Molecular basis of hypertension: role of angiotensinogen. Cell 71: 169-180, 1992

Jones J.M. et al. Adenoviral gene transfer to heart during cardiopulmonary bypass: effect of myocardial protection technique on transgene expression. Eur. J. Cardio-Thorac. Surg. 21: 847-852, 2002

Kaplan N.M.   Primary hypertension: pathogenesis. In: Kaplan N.M Ed. Clinical hypertension. Williams & Wilkins, Baltimore USA, 1998, p. 42

Kato N. et al.   Lack of association between the alpha-adducin locus and essential hypertension in the Japanese population. Hypertension 32: 730-733, 1998

Katritsis D. et al.   Primary restrictive cardiomyopathy: clinical and pathological characteristics. J.Am.Coll.Cardiol. 18: 1230-1235, 1991

Keavney B. et al.   Large-scale test of hypothesized associations between the angiotensin-converting-enzyme insertion/deletion polymorphism and myocardial infarction in about 5,000 cases and 6,000 controls. Lancet 355: 434-442, 2000

Khoo K.L. et al.   Low-density lipoprotein receptor gene mutations in a Southeast Asian population with familial hypercholesterolemia. Clin.Genet. 58: 98-105, 2000

Kipshidze N.N. et al.   Intramural coronary delivery of advanced antisense oligonucleotides reduces neointimal formation in the porcine stent restenosis model. J. Am. Coll. Cardiol, 39: 1686-1691, 2002

Klos K.L. et al.   Genome-wide linkage analysis reveals evidence of multiple regions that influence variation in plasma lipid and apolipoprotein levels associated with risk of coronary heart disease. Arter. Thromb. Vasc.Biol. 21: 971-978, 2001

Koblizek T.I.   Receptor tyrosine kinase signaling in vasculogenesis and angiogenesis. In: "Cardiovascular specific gene expression" P.A. Doevendans, R.S. Reneman and M. van Bilsen Eds., Kluwer Academic Publishers, Dordrecht, The Netherlands, 1999, pp 179-191

Kohl P. et al.   Stretch-induced changes in heart rate and rhythm: clinical observations, experiments and mathematical models. Progr. Biophys. Mol. Biol. 71: 91-138, 1999

Kohl P. et al.   The making of the virtual heart. In: "Vision of the future: Chemistry and Life Science" Thompson J.M.T. Ed. Cambridge University Press, Cambridge 2001, pp 127-149

Kotanko P. et al.   Essential hypertension in African Caribbeans associates with a variant of beta-2 adrenoceptor. Hypertension 30: 773-776, 1997

Kovacs P. et al. Genetic dissection of the syndrome X in the rat. Biochem. Biopys. Res. Commun. 269: 660-665, 2000

Kren V. et al. Genetic isolation of a region of cromosome 8 that exerts major effects on blood pressure and cardiac mass in the spontaneously hypertensive rat. J.Clin.Invest. 99: 577-581, 1997

Kroon A.A. et al. Genetics of hypertension. In " Cardiovascular Genetics for Clinicians" Doevedans P.A. & Wilde A.A.M. Eds. Kluwer Academic Publishers, Dordrecht, The Netherlands, pp.35-49, 2001

Krushkal J. et al. Genotype-wide linkage analyses of systolic blood pressure using discordant siblings. Circulation 99: 1407-1410, 1999

Kushwaha S.S. et al. Restrictive cardiomyopathy. New Engl. J.Med. 336: 267-276, 1997

Lachmeijer A.M.A. et al. A genome-wide scan for pre-ecclampsia in the Netherlands. Eur.J.Hum.Genet. 9: 758-764, 2001

Lander E.S. & Botstein D.S. Homozygosity mapping: a way to map human recessive traits with the DNA of inbred children. Science 236: 1567-1570, 1987

Lander E.S. et al. Initial sequencing and analysis of the human genome. Nature 409 : 860-921, 2001

Lange L.A. et al. Autosomal genome-wide scan for coronary artery calcification in sibships at high risk for hypertension. Atheroscl. Thromb. Vasc. Biol. 22:418-423, 2002

Lessard E. et al. Involvement of CYP2D6 activity in the N-oxydation of procainamide in man. Pharmacogenetics 9: 683-696, 1999

Levy D. et al. Evidence for a gene influencing blood pressure on chromosome 17 – Genome scan linkage results for longitudinal blood pressure phenotypes in subjects from the Framingham Heart Study. Hypertension 36: 477-483, 2000

Li J.J. et al. Comparative study of catheter-mediated gene transfer into heart. Chin.Med.J. 115: 612-613, 2002

Lim D.S. et al. Expression profiling of cardiac genes in human hypertrophic cardiomyopathy: insights into the pathogenesis of phenotypes. J.Am.Coll.Cardiol. 38: 1175-1180, 2001

Luscher T.F. & Noll G. Is it all in the genes? Circulation 99: 2855-2857, 1999

Luther H.P. et al. Analysis of sense and naturally occurring antisense transcripts of myosin heavy chain in the human myocardium. J. Cell. Biochem. 80: 596-605, 2001

MacConnachie A.A. et al. Rapid diagnosis and identification of cross-over sites in patients with glucocorticoid remediable aldosteronism. J.Clin.Endocrin.Metab. 83: 4328-4331, 1998

Mailly F. et al. A common variant in the gene for lipoprotein lipase (Asp9->Asn). Functional implications and prevalence in normal and in hyperlipidemic subjects. Arterioscler. Thromb. Vasc. Biol. 15: 468-478, 1995

Makrill J.J. Protein-protein interactions in intracellular Ca++release channel function. Biochem. J. 337: 345-361, 1999

Marban E. Cardiac channelopathies. Nature 415: 213-218, 2002

Maron B.J. Hypertrophic cardiomyopathy. Lancet 350: 127-133, 1997

McKenna W.J. et al. Diagnosis of Arrhythmogenic Rigt Ventricular Dysplasia/ Cardiomyopathy. Br. Heart J. 71:215-218, 1994

McKoy G. et al. Identification of a deletion in plakoglobin in arrhythmogenic right ventricular cardiomyopathy with palmoplantar keratoderma and woolly hair (Naxos disease). Lancet 355: 2119-2124, 2000

Medley T.L. et al. Fibrillin-1 genotype is associated with aortic stiffness and disease severity in patients with coronary artery disease. Circulation 105: 810-815, 2002

Melacini P. et al. Myocardial involvement is very frequent among patients affected with subclinical Becker muscular dystrophy. Circulation 94: 3168-3195, 1996

Melacini P. et al. Cardiac transplantation in a Duchenne muscular dystrophy carrier. Neuromuscular Disorders 8 : 585-590, 1998

Melacini P. et al. Heart involvement in Muscular Dystrophies due to sarcoglycan gene mutations. Muscle & Nerve 22: 473-479,1999

Mikkelsson J. et al. Platelet glycoprotein Ib alpha HPA-2 Met/VNTR B haplotype as a genetic predictor of myocardial infarction and sudden cardiac death. Circulation 104: 876-880, 2001

Milasin J. et al. A point mutation in the 5' splice site of the dystrophin gene first intron responsible for X-linked dilated cardiomyopathy. Hum.Molec.Genet. 5: 73-79, 1996

Miserez A.R. et al. High prevalence of familial defective apolipoprotein B-100 in Switzerland. J. Lipid Res. 35: 574-583, 1994

Muntoni F. et al. Deletion of the dystrophin muscle-promoter region associated with X-linked dilated cardiomyopathy. New Engl.J.Med. 329: 921-925, 1993

Nakagawa K. & Ishizaki T. Therapeutical relevance of pharmacogenetic factors in cardiovascular medicine. Pharmacol. & Therapeut. 86: 1-28, 2000

Nebert D.W. Pharmacogenetics and pharmacogenomics: why is this relevant to the clinical geneticist? Clin. Genet. 56: 247-258, 1999

Olivieri O. et al. Homozygosity for angiotensinogen 235T variant increases the risk of myocardial infarction in patients with multi-vessel coronary artery disease. J. Hypertens. 19: 879-884, 2001

Olivieri O. et al. Different impact of deletion polymorphism of gene on the risk of renal and coronary artery disease. J. Hypertens. 20: 37-43, 2002

Okubo K. et al. Large scale cDNA sequencing for analysis of quantitative and qualitative aspects of gene expression. Nature genetics 2 : 173-179, 1992

Ortiz-Lopez R. et al. Evidence for a dystrophin missense mutation as a cause of X-linked dilated cardiomyopathy. Circulation 95: 2434-2440, 1997

Pankow J.S. Possible locus on chromosome 18q influencing postural systolic blood pressure changes. Hypertension 36: 471-476, 2000

Pastinen T. et al. Minisequencing: a specific tool for DNA analysis and diagnostics on oligonucleotide arrays. Genome Res. 7: 606-614, 1997

Perola M. et al. Genome-wide scan of predisposing loci for increased diastolic blood pressure in Finnish siblings. J. Hypertens. 18: 1579-1585, 2000

194

Poch E. et al.   G-Protein beta-3 subunit gene variant and left ventricular hypertrophy in essential hypertension. Hypertension 35: 214-218, 2000

Podlowski S. et al. Cardiac Troponin I sense-antisense RNA duplexes in the myocardium. J. Cell. Biochem. 85: 198-207, 2002

Pravenec M. et al. Genetic analysis of cardiovascular risk factor clustering in spontaneous hypertension. Folia Biol. 46: 233-240, 2000

Priori S.G. et al. Genetic and molecular basis of cardiac arrhythmias: impact on clinical management. Parts I and II. Circulation 99: 518-528, 1999

Priori S.G. et al. Genetic and molecular basis of cardiac arrhythmias: impact on clinical management. Part III. Circulation 99: 674-681, 1999

Priori S.G. et al. Mutations in the cardiac ryanodine receptor gene (hRyR2) underlie catecholaminergic polymorphic ventricular tachycardia. Circulation 103: 196-2000, 2001

Rankinen T. et al.   Genomic scan for exercise blood pressure in the Health, Risk factors, Exercise training and Genetics (HERITAGE) family study. Hypertension 38: 30-37, 2001

Rice T. et al.   Genome-wide linkage analysis of systolic and diastolic blood pressure. The Quebec Family study. Circulation 102: 1956, 2000

Roberts R. & Brugada R.   Genetic aspects of arrhythmias. Am.J.Med.Genet. 97: 310-318, 2000

Schena M. et al.   Quantitative monitoring of gene expression patterns with a complementary DNA microarray. Science 270: 467-470, 1995

Schwartz P.J. et al.   A molecular link between the sudden infant death syndrome and the long-QT syndrome. N.Engl.J.Med. 343: 262-267, 2000

Sehl P.D. et al. Application of cDNA microarrays in determining molecular phenotype in cardiac growth, development and response to injury. Circulation 101: 1990-1999, 2000

Sellers K.W. et al.   Gene therapy to control hypertension: current studies and future perspectives. Am. J. Med. Sci. 322: 1-6, 2001

Seidman J.G. & Seidman C.   The genetic basis for cardiomyopathy: from mutation identification to mechanistic paradigm. Cell 104: 557-567, 2001

Senti M. et al. Physical activity modulates the combined effect of a common variant of the lipoprotein lipase gene and smoking on serum triglyceride levels and high-density lipoprotein cholesterol in men. Hum.Genet. 109: 385-392, 2001

Singer D.R.J. et al. Angiotensin-converting enzyme polymorphism: what to do anout all the confusion? Circulation 94: 236-239, 1996

Sivo Z. et al. Accelerated congenics for mapping two blood pressure quantitative loci on chromosome 10 of Dahl rats. J. Hypertens. 20. 45-53, 2002

Soro A. et al. Genome scans provide evidence for Low-HDL-C loci on chromosomes 8q23, 16q24.1.q24.2 and 20q13.11 in Finnish families. Am.J.Hum.Genet. 70: 1333-1340, 2002

Spielman R.S. et al. Transmission test for linkage disequilibrium: the insulin gene region and insulin-dependent diabetes mellitus (IDDM). Am.J. Hum. Genet. 52: 506-516, 1993

Splering W. et al. Sensitivity, but not reactivity to angiotensin II is associated with angiotensin II type 1 receptor A1166C polymorphism. Hypertension 36: 411-416, 2000

Spiridonova M.G. Analysis of gene complexes predisposing to coronary atherosclerosis. Russian J. Genet. 38: 300-308, 2002

Stein Y. et al. Is there a genetic basis for resistance to atherosclerosis? Atherosclerosis 160: 1-10, 2002

Stanton L.W. et al. Altered patterns of gene expression in response to myocardial infarction. Circ.Res. 86: 939-945, 2000

Sullivan J.L. Iron and the genetics of cardiovascular disease. Circulation 100: 1260 1263, 1999

Svetkcy L.P. et al. Association of hypertension with beta-2 and alpha-2 adrenergic receptor genotype. Hypertension 27: 1210-1215, 1996

Swynghedauw B. Molecular Cardiology for the Cardiologist. Kluwer Academic Publishers, Boston, 1998, pp.170-211

Swynghedauw B. Susceptibility-conferring polymorphic genotypes in cardiovascular multifactorial syndromes. Eur. Heart J. 23: 271-273, 2002

Taal M.W. et al. Angiotensin-converting enzyme gene polymorphism in renal disease: clinically relevant? Curr.Opin.Nephrol.Hypertens. 9: 651-657, 2000

Thiene G. et al. Arrhythmogenic right ventricular cardiomyopathy. Trends Cardiovasc.Med. 7: 84-90, 1997

Tiso N. et al. Identification of mutations in the cardiac ryanodine receptor gene in families affected with arrhythmogenic right ventricular cardiomyopathy type 2. Hum. Molec. Genet. 10: 189-194, 2001

Towbin J.A. et al. X-linked dilated cardiomyopathy: molecular genetic evidence of linkage to the Duchenne muscular dystrophy (dystrophin) gene at the Xp21 locus. Circulation 87: 1854-1865, 1993

Towbin J.A. Molecular genetic basis of sudden cardiac death. Cardiovascular Pathology 10: 283-295, 2001

Towbin J.A. & Bowles N.E. The failing heart. Nature 145: 227-233,2002

Van Geel P.P. et al. Angiotensin II type 1 receptor A1166C gene polymorphism is associated with an increased response to angiotensin II in human arteries. Hypertension 35: 717-721, 2000

Velculescu V.E. et al. Serial analysis of gene expression. Science 270: 484-487, 1995

Venter J.C. et al. The sequence of the human genome. Science 291: 1304-1351, 2001

Weiss R.H. & Randour C.J. Attenuation of matrix protein secretion by antisense oligodeoxynucleotides to the cyclin kinase inhibitor p21(Waf1/Cip1). Atherosclerosis 161: 105-112, 2002

Ward K. et al. A molecular variant of angiotensinogen associated with preeclampsia. Nat.Genet. 4: 59-61, 1993

Weeks D.E. & Lange K. A multilocus extension of the affected pedigree member method of linkage analysis. Am.J.Hum.Genet. 50: 859-868, 1992

Wilkins M.R. et al. Pharmacogenetis and the treatment of cardiovascular disease. Heart 84: 353-354, 2000

Winslow R.L. et al. Computational models of the failing myocyte: relating altered gene expression to cellular function. Philosph. Transact. Royal Soc. UK, Series A, 359: 1187-1200, 2001

Winslow R.L. et al. Mapping, modelling and visual exploration of structure-functions relationships in the heart. IBM Syst.J. 40: 342-359, 2001

Woosley R.L. & Roden D.M. Pharmacologic causes of arrhythmogenic actions of antiarrythmic drugs. Am. J. Cardiol. 59: 19E-25E, 1987

Wu K.K. et al. Thrombomodulin Ala455Val polymorphism and risk of coronary heart disease. Circulation 103: 1386-1389, 2001

Zhu D.L. et al. Linkage of hypertension to chromosome 2q14-q23 in Chinese families. J.Hypertens. 19: 55-61, 2001

GLOSSARY

ALLELE: a gene variant showing a frequency of at least 1% in a given human population. There may be several alleles for a single gene, but in a single individual there are two alleles, each on one of the homologous chromosomes

AMPLICON: product of PCR amplification

AMPLIFICATION: production of a large number of copies of a given DNA segment

ANEUPLOID: abnormal number of chromosomes in a karyotype, due to presence or absence of single chromosomes

ANIMAL MODEL: animal showing a disease mimicking or reproducing a human disorder; it may be produced by mutation or by sophisticated techniques of manipulation and gene transfer

ASSORTMENT: random distribution of parental chromosomes to gametes; genes carried by different chromosomes undergo independent segregation, while genes carried by the same chromosomes tend to be transmitted in linkage

AUTOSOME: any chromosome in the karyotype, except X-chromosome, Y-chromosome and mitochondrial DNA

BP: stands for "base pair"; synonym: nt, nucleotide

CANDIDATE: this term applies to a gene or to a chromosomal region; in search of the gene involved in a given disease, the first step is usually to discriminate between candidate chromosomal regions (by linkage analysis); the second step, once identified the chromosomal region, is to discriminate between different candidate genes, by screening each of them for possible causative mutations

CARRIER: a person carrying in his DNA a mutant copy of a given gene, in heterozygosis

c-DNA: stands for "complementary DNA"; DNA obtained by reverse transcription on a mRNA template

CENTROMERE: part of the chromosome involved in attachment to mitotic or meiotic spindle. Each chromosome pair is characterized by position of centromere, which defines the length of chromosomal arms

CHIMERA: individual made by cells derived from two different zygotes; artificial chimeras may be created, by manipulation of blastocysts

CHIMERIC GENE: abnormal gene obtained by fusion of DNA sequences originally belonging to two different genes

CHROMATID: one of the two double-stranded DNA copies of chromosomal DNA, resulting after DNA replication; at metaphase of cell division each chromosome is longitudinally subdivided into two sister chromatids, interconnected in correspondence of the centromere

CHROMATIN: old-fashioned name indicating chromosomal material which can be stained in the nucleus during interphase. Cytologists identified "euchromatin" as a main constituent of chromosomes, in contrast to "heterochromatin", which appears in dense masses in interphase nuclei, but disappears at the beginning of meiosis or mitosis

CODON: a triplet made by contiguous nucleotides, specifying a given aminoacid or a stop

COMPOUND HETEROZYGOTE: an individual carrying two different mutations of the same gene; he will be heterozygote for each of the two mutations

CONGENITAL: manifested at birh

CONSANGUINEOUS, MARRIAGE: between blood relatives, usually between first cousins or between uncle and niece

CONSENSUS SEQUENCE: part of a DNA sequence, identified as a typical sequence

CONTIGUOUS GENE DELETION SYNDROME: Syndrome due to deletion of a chromosomal segment including different genes. Deletion of an X-chromosome segment is pathogenic in males, since they have only one X-chromosome; deletion of an autosomal segment may be pathogenic because of dosage effects or because some mutations, originally carried in heterozygosis, become uncompensated by loss of their respectively normal alleles

CROSSING-OVER: cytogenetical appearance of the exchange of chromosomal segments between chromatids of two homologous chromosomes, at meiotic prophase

DIPLOID: an organism or cell showing two sets of chromosomes

DNA ARRAY: a series of arrayed oligonucleotides or of cDNAs fixed on a glass or plastic slide; DNA arrays are used in hybridization assays, for different purposes (mutation detection, linkage analysis, expression profiling)

DNA CHIP: the principle of this techology is the same applied to DNA arrays and micro-arrays, with the difference that microarrays are usually prepared in individual research laboratories, whereas DNA-chips are industrial products

DNA SEQUENCING: analysis of the sequence of a given segment of DNA molecule, producing as output the ordered series of constituent nucleotides; DNA sequencing is presently performed by automated apparatuses, based on capillary electrophoresis.

DOMINANT: inherited trait which is manifested in the heterozygote

DOMINANT NEGATIVE MUTATION: a mutation which, in heterozygosis, results in an altered function and which negatively interferes with the function of the normal allele

DOUBLE HETEROZYGOTE: individual in heterozygosis for mutations in two different genes

DYNAMIC MUTATION: mutational alteration of a DNA sequence, which undergoes modification through subsequent generations; a typical example is given by triplet repeat expansions

ECTOPIC EXPRESSION: Abnormal expression of a given gene in tissue(s) where it is normally unexpressed

EPIGENETIC: any factor capable of affecting phenotype, with no modification of genotype

ES CELLS: stands for "Embryonic Stem cells"

EST: Expressed Sequence Tag; segment of cDNA corresponding to an expressed gene in a given cell or tissue.

EUPLOID: the correct chromosome number for a given individual or species. In humans euploidy corresponds to 46 chromosomes in diploid cells and 23 chromosomes in haploid cells

EXON: intragenic DNA segment included in the primary transcript and in mature mRNA; the corresponding genetic information is translated into an aminoacid sequence

EXPANSION: increase in number of triplet repeats

EXPRESSIVITY: degree of variability of phenotypic expression; genes may show constant or variable expressivity

FRAME-SHIFT MUTATION: a deletion or insertion of nucleotides altering the correct series of codons and consequently disrupting the reading frame

GAMETE: specialized cell participating in fertilization

GAIN-OF-FUNCTION: type of mutation characterized by increase in one or more function of a given protein. The same term, imprecisely used, indicates the gain of a completely novel property (novel property mutation)

GENE TARGETING: artificial modification of a given gene within a living cell, usually obtained by gene transfer followed by recombination

GENE TRANSFER: transfer of a DNA sequence (corresponding to a selected gene) into a living cell, by means of artificial carriers (vectors) or by cell manipulations

GENETIC HETEROGENEITY: situation in which a single phenotype may be genetically determined by mutation in different genes (locus heterogeneity)

GENOME: the total genetic complement of a given organism, cell or virus; the complement includes both coding sequences and non-coding sequences

GENOME SCAN: linkage analysis of a given phenotype, by testing association with each of a large series of markers, distributed along all chromosomes of a given genome. In humans, a "dense" genome scan usually involves linkage analysis with about 800 DNA markers; synonym: genome-wide search

GENOMICS: a novel discipline, investigating structure ("structural genomics") and function ("functional genomics") of genomes

GENOTYPE: this term equally applies to the genetic constitution of a single individual and to the kind of alleles carried by a single individual at a given locus or at different loci

GERM CELLS: cells involved in production of gametes

HAPLOID: individual or cell carrying only one set of chromosomes; gametes are haploid

HAPLOINSUFFICIENCY: when a mutation in heterozygosis produces phenotypic effects

HAPLOTYPE: the series of alleles of adjacent genes in a given chromosome; two homologous chromosomal segment usually show different haplotypes

HEMIZYGOSITY: condition due to presence of a single cromosome, instead of two; emizygosity is typical in males for X-linked genes: since each X-linked gene is in single copy, there cannot be either homozygosity, or heterozygosity, but hemizygosity

HETEROCHROMATIN: type of nuclear chromatin, characterized by persistence of spiralization during interphase and by late DNA replication; genes within heterochromatic segments are usually not transcribed

HETEROZYGOSIS: situation in which the two homologous of a single locus carry two different alleles (e.g. one normal and one mutant allele); the individual showing this situation is said to be "heterozygote" at this locus, or "heterozygous" for the mutation

HOMOLOGOUS CHROMOSOMES: chromosomes belonging to the same pair in the chromosome set of a cell or of an organism; homologous chromosomes show the same series of loci

HOMOLOGOUS RECOMBINATION: recombination between homologous DNA sequences, this phenomenon occurs regularly at meiosis between segments of homologous chromosomes; homologous recombination may occur also between a chromosomal DNA sequence and a foreign DNA showing partial homology, as in gene targeting

HOMOZYGOSITY: condition of having two identical alleles (copies of the same gene) at a given locus

HOUSEKEEPING GENES: genes coding for products which are believed to be needed by all cell types in a given organism

HYBRIDIZATION: bonding of two segments of nucleic acids (DNA-DNA or DNA-RNA), thanks to the complementarity of nucleotide sequences; in case of perfect complementarity, the "hybrid" will be stable and relatively resistant to heat denaturation, while imperfect complementarity produce instability and proneness to denaturation by heat

INCIDENCE RATE: rate at wich a given disease is manifested in a given series of births

INDEX CASE: the first case affected with a given disease known in a given family; index case is the starting point for reconstructing the family tree and the family history for the disease

INFORMATIVITY : (of a meiose, of a family) possibility to follow the segregation of a given DNA marker

INTRON: intragenic segment of DNA included in the primary transcript, but subsequently removed by splicing, during mRNA maturation process

ISOLATED CASE: a single case affected with a specific disease, occurring in a family with negative history for the same disorder; an isolated case may result from novel mutation, but, more frequently, it may result from normal segregation in a family showing sibships of small size in previous generations

KARYOTYPE: the set of chromosomes characteristic of a species, of a single individual or of a single cell. Human normal karyotype corresponds to a set of 23 pairs of homologues, 46 chromosomes in total

KILOBASE: 1,000 nucleotides

LINKAGE: non-random segregation of genes, due to their vicinity on the same chromosome; linkage may be broken only by meiotic recombination (crossing-over)

LINKAGE DISEQUILIBRIUM: occurrence of specific haplotypes at higher (or lower) frequency than expected

LINKAGE MAP: a chromosome map in which position of single genes is reconstructed on the basis of their reciprocal recombination frequency; genes showing low recombination frequency are close, those showing very low recombination or no recombination at all are very close to each other

LOCUS: a given place in a given chromosome; in the past "locus" was often a synonym of "gene", since it was the "place" of the gene on the chromosome

LOCUS HETEROGENEITY: see genetic heterogeneity

LOD SCORE: literally: "Log Of the Odds score"; it measures the probability that the observed distribution of genotypes in a given family, in respect to two variable traits (e.g. a disease locus and a DNA marker locus) might be due to linkage between the two considered loci; higher the value of the lod score, lower will be the probability that the observed association is due to chance

MARKER: a polymorphic DNA sequence or protein, which might be used for following the segregation of the given chromosome or chromosomal segment where the corresponding locus is placed; DNA markers are extensively used in mapping disease genes, in paternity testing and in forensic medicine

MEGABASE: 1,000,000 nucleotides

MEIOSIS: type of cell division leading to the production of haploid gametes; it is characterized by two subsequent cell divisions without DNA replication and by a long-lasting prophase of the first division, where recombination between homologous chromosomes takes place

MENDELIAN TRAIT: a trait inherited according to the rules originally proposed by Mendel

MISSENSE: mutation leading to an aminoacid substitution

MICROSATELLITE: see STRS

MITOCHONDRIAL DNA: Circular double-stranded DNA carried by mitochondria. It includes 37 genes, including those encoding mitochondrial rRNAs and tRNAs

MONOSOMY: presence of a single copy of a given chromosome; most monosomies in humans are lethal before birth

MOSAICISM: presence of two or more different cell lineages in the same individual

MULTIFACTORIAL INHERITANCE: genetic determination of a trait, due to cooperative effect of several genes and by the effect of environmental factors

MUTATION: any change in a DNA molecule, due to replicative errors or to the effect of chemical or physical mutagenic interactions

MUTATION RATE: rate at which mutation occurs; mutation rate is symbolized by μ ; essentially, $\mu = n/N$, where n is the number of mutant copies of DNA and N is the total number of copies

MUTATION SCREENING: systematic investigation for detection of mutations in a given segment of DNA

NONSENSE: mutation producing a stop codon

NT: stands for "nucleotide"

OBLIGATE CARRIER: individual for whom heterozygosity for a given allele may be establish, regardless its phenotype (e.g. because he/she have a father and a son both showing the phenotype corresponding to the considered allele)

OLIGO: stands for OLIGONUCLEOTIDE; a short (usually from 8 to 50nt) DNA sequence used as a DNA probe or as PCR primer

PCR: Polymerase Chain Reaction; a simple method for amplifying a selected DNA segment

PEDIGREE: the family tree

PENETRANCE, REDUCED: when a given phenotype is not manifested by all individuals carrying the same allele determining the considered trait

PHARMACOGENETICS: discipline investigating on interindividual differences in response to administration of specific drugs

PHARMACOGENOMICS: a novel dicipline focused on search of novel pharmacogenetic variants, by exploiting genomic information

PHASE: situation of "coupling" or "repulsion" of mutant alleles in two loci belonging to a given chromosomal segment

PHENOCOPY: a phenotype apparently corresponding to the effect of mutation in a given gene, but in reality due to environmental effects

PHENOTYPE: the observed characteristics of a given individual

PLEIOTROPY: multiple effects (e.g. pathogenic effects in different tissues) produced by a single gene mutation

POINT MUTATION: a mutation involving a single nucleotide or a small number of nucleotides

POLYGENIC: due to cooperative effect of several genes

POLYMORPHISM: occurrence of two or more alleles (polymorphic variants) in a given population. A locus is considered polymorphic when its rarest variant shows in the population a frequency of 1% or higher

POSITIONAL CLONING: identification of a gene, starting from information on its chromosomal location, in the absence of prior knowledge of its product

PREVALENCE RATE: rate of occurrence of a given disease in a given population sample

PRIMER: a short oligonucleotide used for priming the reaction of DNA synthesis by DNA polymerase (in Polymerase Chain Reaction)

PROBAND: a person whose status (affected, carrier, non-affected) is to be defined

PROBE: a DNA or RNA sequence, used to detect the precence of a complementary sequence by molecular hybridization; to this purpose, probe is usually radioactively or fluorescently labelled

PROTEOMICS: field of present biochemical research, dealing with comprehensive analysis and cataloguing of structures and functions of all proteins of a given cell or tissue

PSEUDOGENE: a functionally inactive gene in the genome; pseudogenes may derive from mutational inactivation of a member of a gene family, or by retrotransposition.

QANTITATIVE TRAIT: a biological characteristics showing a continuous variation among phenotypes (e.g. body weight), in contrast with Mendelian traits which show a discrete variation. Since quantitative traits are determined by several genes, they show polygenic inheritance

QTL: Quantitative Trait Locus. A locus corresponding to a gene involved in determination of a quantitative trait

RECOMBINANT DNA: technology based on cutting DNA by restriction enzymes and inserting the resulting DNA segment in a foreign DNA

RECOMBINATION: formation of new combinations of segments of chromosomal DNA, due to reciprocal exchange between homologous chromosomes (see also crossing-over)

RECURRENCE RISK: probability that a given inherited disease, observed in a family, will be manifested by another member of the family in the same or in a subsequent generation

RESTRICTION ENZYMES: bacterial endonucleases recognizing specific sites (usually short palyndromes) within a DNA sequence; they cleave the DNA molecule within recognition site or nearby

RISK-ALLELE: a gene variant associated with a specific disease

RT-PCR: PCR amplification on cDNAs obtained by reverse transcription from mRNAs extracted from a given tissue sample; this method is routinely used to quick check the expression of given gene in a given tissue, by using gene-specific PCR primers

SEGREGATION: separation of chromosomes of each pair; by consequence, separation of the two alleles of each gene carried by the considered chromosome

SIBSHIP: all siblings (brothers and/or sisters) in a given family

SIGNAL TRANSDUCTION: a multistep process by which perturbation of the extracellular or intracellular environment is "sensed" at genomic level and it is followed by response in terms of activation or repression of specific genes

SILENT MUTATION: a single-nucleotide substitution in a codon, resulting in a synonymous codon (i.e. specifying the same aminoacid)

SNP: Single Nucleotide Polymorphism; a polymorphism in a DNA sequence, due to variation in a single nucleotide

SOMATIC CELLS: cells of a given organism, not involved in transmission of genetic information to the following generation

SOUTHERN BLOT: a clever method devised in 1975 by E.M. Southern, for transferring onto nitrocellulose sheets ("filter") DNA molecules separated by agarose gel electrophoresis; this method opened the way to development of human molecular genetics. The same principle, applied to transfer of electrophoretically separated RNAs and proteins is named "Northern blot" and "Western blot", respectively.

SPLICING: excision of intronic sequences from the primary transcript

SPORADIC CASE: an isolated case showing a Mendelian disease trait, due to new mutation

STRP: Short Tandem Repeat Polymorphism; variable number of tandemly repeated bi-tri- or tetra-nucleotide units, at a given locus, aliases: VNTR, Microsatellite

STOP CODON: A nonsense codon, showing no correspondence with any tRNA and, hence, with any aminoacid

SUSCEPTIBILITY LOCUS: a locus including a gene conferring to the individual increased risk of developing a given disease

SYNONYMOUS: literally: with the same meaning; it applies to codons specifying the same aminoacid

TELOMERE: the tip of each chromosome end; abbreviation: *tel*

TRANSCRIPT: mRNA molecule, produced by transcription

TRANSCRIPTION: transfer of genetic information from one DNA strand to a mRNA sequence, operated by RNA polymerase

TRANSFECTION: transfer of a foreign gene (transgene) in a target cell

TRANSGENIC: organism carrying a foreign gene, artificially introduced in its genome; transgenic animals are often produced for obtaining animal models of human diseases

TRANSLATION: process by which coded genetic information, transcribed from DNA to mRNA, is then translated into an aminoacid sequence, by aid of the ribosomal protein synthesis machinery

TRANSPOSON: a DNA segment capable of self replication and of insertion in a different location in the genome

TRIPLET EXPANSION: increase in number of triplet repeats, through subsequent generations. Very long stretches of triplets may result, which in some cases are pathogenic

TRISOMY: presence of three homologous chromosomes, in place of the normal pair; this abnormality produces complex phenotypes; the most common trisomy in humans is Down syndrome (trisomy of chromosome 21)

VNTR: Variable Number of Tandem Repeats; series of tandemly repeated oligo- or poly-nucleotides within DNA sequences; this term includes microsatellites, minisatellites and megasatellites, but it is mostly used to indicate minisatellites (STRP, see)

X-LINKED: carried by X-chromosome; mutations in X-linked genes produce X-linked diseases

ZYGOTE: diploid cell resulting from fusion of male and female gametes

APPENDIX I

UPDATED INFORMATION FROM THE WEB

The development of Internet made accessible on public domain an unbelievable mass of data. However, relatively few websites provide reliable and permanently updated information, quick and easy access, proper links to other websites and the possibility of dowloading documents or printing single webpages.

The Reader will found below a handful of web addresses, which may be confidently used as reference sites or as starting points for navigation in the web.

Cardiovascular Diseases

http:www.mic.ki.se/Diseases/c14.html

The website is maintained by Karolinska Intitute Library, (Stockholm, Sweden). It is a collection of links to websites dealing with heart and vascular diseases

OMIM

http://www.ncbi.nlm.nlh.gov./omim/

Originally developed at the John Hpkins University, it is presently maintained by NCBI (National Center for Biological Information).

This searchable database is the most valuable source for quick information on different aspects of genetic diseases.

GENECARD

http://www.cgd.icnet.uk/genecards/

This searchable database, developed at the Weizmann Institute (Rehovot, Israel), provides updated information on human genes and proteins. The search may start also by typing the name of a given disease. Each "card" have links to OMIM and to different genomic databases

LOCUSLINK

http://www.ncbi.nlm.nih.gov/LocusLink/index.html

This is the core of the databases maintained at NCBI, centered on human genes. Each entry have multiple links to different databases, enabling the retrieval of all available information, from DNA sequence to papers in the literature

PUBMED

http:// www.ncbi.nlm.nih.gov/PubMed/

This website enables the Reader to retrieve a series of titles and abstracts pertaining a selected subject. Titles and abtracts can be printed; for some papers, download of full text is permitted.

HUMAN GENOME BROWSER

http://genome.ucsc.edu/

This website provides direct "views" on segments of the human genome, simply by typing names of genes or of DNA markers. Graphics enables to see placement, size and internal organization of genes. Each "object" on the string is directely linked to pertinent database(s). This complicated interface was developed in few months of restless work by a small team, leaded by Jim Kent, at the University of California, Santa Cruz. The harsh competition with scientists working at Celera Genomics ended with the historical announcement of the first released draft of human genome, jointly given by the private company Celera Genomics and by the public Consortium.

OMIM IDs CORRESPONDING TO MONOGENIC DISORDERS RELEVANT TO CARDIOLOGY

OMIM (On-line Mendelian Inheritance in Man) is the main reference database for human genes involved in disease phenotypes. It is permanently updated and accessible on public domain at website http://www.ncbi.nlm.nih.gov./omim/

In following pages, an index of monogenic diseases of cardiological interest is provided, reporting for each entry, the corresponding OMIM number, for quick accession to the database.

For most entries, mode of inheritance of the disease may be inferred from corresponding OMIM number. Numbers starting with 1 refer to diseases with autosomal dominant inheritance (entries created before May 15, 1994); those starting with 2 refer to autosomal recessives (entries created before May 15, 1994). Entries which number starts with 3 and 4 refers to diseases inherited respectively as X-linked or Y-linked traits. Numbers starting with 5 refer to diseases showing mitochondrial (mtDNA) inheritance, while those starting with 6 refer to autosomal loci, diseases or phenotypes included in the catalogue after May 15, 1994.

Adrenal hyperplasia V Syndrome	202110
Alagille syndrome	118450
Aldosteronism, Glucocorticoid-remediable GRA	103900
Aminoglycoside-induced deafness	561000
Amyloidosis, Familial, Finnish type	137350
Apparent Mineralcorticoid Excess Syndrome AME	218030
Apolipoprotein B100, defective, familial	107730
Arrhythmia	115000
Arteries fibromuscular dysplasia	135580
ARVD1	107970
ARVD2	600996
ARVD3	602086
ARVD4	602087
ARVD5	604400
ARVD6	604401
ARVD7	125647
Asplenia and Polysplenia	208530
Atrial cardiomyopathy with heart block	108770
Atrial fibrillation with bradyarrhythmia	163800
Atrial septal defect	108800
Atrial septal defect and AV conduction defect	108900
Atrial septal defect, secundum, with various defects	603642
Atrial tachyarrhythmia with short PR interval	108950
Atrioventricular dissociation	209600
Atrio-ventricular septal defect	600309
Bardet-Biedl Syndrome BBS2	606151
Bardet-Biedl Syndrome BBS4	600374

Barth's syndrome	302060
Brugada syndrome	601144
Cardiomyopathy with Microcephaly	251220
Cardiomyopathy, congestive, with hypogonadism	212112
Cardiomyopathy and cataract	212350
Cardiomyopathy, fatal fetal, myocardial	606163
Cardiomyopathy, infantine histiocytoid	500000
Cardiomyopathy-hypogonadism-collagenoma	115250
Cardioneuromyopathy, hyaline masses,nemaline	606842
Cardioskelctal Desmin-related myopathy	601419
Char syndrome	169100
CMD pure (?)	212110
CMD1A	115200
CMD1B	600884
CMD1C	601493
CMD1D	601494
CMD1E	601154
CMD1F	602067
CMD1G	604145
CMD1H	604288
CMD1I	604765
CMD1J	605362
CMD1K	605582
CMD1L	606685
CMD3A	300069
CMH/WPW	600858
CMH1	192600
CMH2	115195

CMH3	115196
CMH4	115197
CMH5	115198
CMH6	600858
CMH7	191044
CMH8	160790
CMH9	188840
CoA dehydrogenase, very long chain, deficiency	201475
Conduction defect, with sudden death	115080
DiGeorge syndrome	188400
Distichiasis, cardiac congenital anomalies	126320
Duchenne and Becker muscular dystrophy	300377
Ebstein anomaly	224700
Ehlers-Danlos syndrome	130000
Emery-Dreyfuss muscular dystrophy	310300
Fabry's disease	301500
Fibromuscular dysplasia of arteries	135580
Gordon's Syndrome	145260
Heart block, congenital	234700
Heart block , progressive, familial, Type I	113900
Heart block , progressive, familial, Type I.I	604559
Heart block, progressive, familial, Type II	140400
Heart-hand syndrome, Spanish type	140450
Holt-Oram syndrome	142900
Hypercholesterolemia, familial	143890
Hypercholesterolemia, familial, type 2	603813
Hypercholesterolemia, familial, type 3	603776
Hypertension, dominant, with early onset	600983

Hypertension, essential	145500
Jervell and Lange-Nielsen syndrome	220400
Left ventricular noncompaction	606617
Left ventricular noncompaction, congenital defects	601239
Left ventricular noncompaction, isolated, familial	604169
Leigh syndrome	256000
Leopard syndrome	151100
Liddle Syndrome	177200
LQT1	192500
LQT2	152427
LQT3	603830
LQT4	600919
LQT5	176261
LQT6	603796
Malignant hyperthermia, susceptibility	145600
Marfan's syndrome	154700
MERRF (Myoclonic Epilepsy with Ragged Red	590060
Muscular dystrophy, limb-girdle	15900
Myotonic dystrophy	160900
Myxoma, familial (Carney complex)	160980
Myxoma, intracardiac	255960
Naxos disease	188840
Nodal rythm	163800
Noonan's syndrome	163950
Pseudoxantoma elasticum	264800
Cardiomyopathy, restrictive	115210
Sinus Arrhythmia, phocomelia-ectrodactyly	171480
Situs inversus viscerum	270100

Tachyarrhythmia with short PR interval	108950
Tachycardia, hypertension, microphtalmos	272550
Tetralogy of Fallot	187500
Velocardiofacial syndrome	192430
Ventricular extrasystoles, syncope, Robin yndrome	192445
Ventricular fibrillation, paroxysmal, familial	603829
Ventricular tachycardia, familial	192605
Ventricular tachycardia, stress-induced	604772
William syndrome	194050
Wolff-Parkinson White syndrome	194200

GENES ENCODING IONIC CHANNELS AND EXPRESSED IN HUMAN HEART

Genes reportedly expressed only in the heart are indicated in bold; asterisk (*) indicates that mutation of the channel causes a cardiac disease; column three reports additional tissue(s) in which a given channel is expressed (AD: adipose tissue; AO: aorta; B: Brain; COL: colon; CHO: choclea; EY: eye; FI: fibroblasts; I: ileus; KD: Kidney; LI: Liver; LU: Lung; PA: pancreas; PL: placenta; RT: retina; SC: spinal cord; SG: salivary gland; SKM: skeletal muscle; SM: smooth muscle; SP: spleen; T: testis; THY: thymus; TR: trachea; UT: uterus; V: vascular endothelium)

CHANNEL	CODE	EXPRESSION	LOCUS
Cl-	CLC-4	SKM, B, KD,RT	1p13.3
Cl-	CLIC4	B,PL, SKM	1p36.11
Na+	**SCN5A ***		3p21
Na+	SCN7A	UT, SKM	2q21-q23
Na+	SCN1B	B,SKM	19q13.12
Ca2+	CACNA1C	LU,SM, FI	12p13.33
Ca2+	CACNA2D1	SKM, B, I	7q21.11
Ca2+	CACNB1	SKM, B, SP	17q21.1
Ca2+	CACNB2	B,LU, AO	10p12.33
Ca2+	**RYR2 ***		1q43
Ca2+ATPase	ATP2A2 SERCA2a	SKM	12q24.11
K+	**KCNA5**		12p13.32
K+	KCND2	B, AO	7q31.31
K+	**KCND3**		1p13.3
K+	KCNE2 *	B, SKM, PA, PL, KD, COL, THY	21q22.12
K+	KCNE1L	SKM,B, SC, PL	Xq23
K+	KCNF1	B	2p25.1

K+	**KCNG2**		18q23
K+	KCNQ1 *	PA,CHO	11p15.4
K+ 4x> Na+	HCN2	B	19p13.3
K+ 4x> Na+	HCN4	B, T	15q24.1
K+	KCNJ2 *	B, SKM, LU, KD, PL	17q24.3
K+	**KCNJ3**		2q24.1
K+	KCNJ4	SKM,B	22q13.1
K+	KCNJ5	PA	11q24.3
K+	**KCNH2 ***		7q36.1
K+	KCNN1	B	19p13.11
K+	KCNN3	B,SKM,LI	1q23.1
K+	**SUR2A**		12p12.1
Cat Chn	CNGA3	T, KD, EY	2q11.2
Na-K-Cl co-tr	SLC12A6	V, B,SKM,KD	15q14
Na-K-Cl co-tr	SLC12A7	KD	5p15.33
Cat Chn	TRPC2	T,B	
Cat Chn	TRPC3	B, PL, SKM	4q27
Cat Chn	TRPC7	LU, B, SM, EY	21q22.3
Cat Chn	TRPV4	B, LI, KD, AD, T, SG, TR	12q24.1
Cat Chn	TRPM7	KD, LI, SP, LU, B	15q21

(by courtesy of Dr. C. Veronese)

CREDITS

Some illustrations of this book are modifications of figures which were previously published in books or in scientific journals.

In particular:

Figures 1,1, 1.5, 1.6, 1.7, 1.8 and 2.6 were from Strachan T. : "The human genome" Bios Scientific Publishers, Oxford (UK), 1992

Figures 4.4 and 4.5 from Strachan T. and Read A.P.: "Human Molecular Genetics", Bios Scientific Publishers, Oxford (UK), 1999

Figure 1.2 was from McKonkey E.H. : "Human Genetics" Jones & Bartlett Publ. Boston (USA), 1993

Figure 1.4 was from Modrek B. & Lee C.: A genomic view of alternative splicing. Nature Genetics 30: 13-18, 2002

Figure 2.7 was from Werner T. : Models for prediction and recognition of eukaryotic promoters. Mamm.Genome 10: 168-175, 1999

Figure 2.9 was from Albert R. et al: Error and attack tolerance of complex networks. Nature 406: 378-382, 2000

Figure 3.16 was from Marian A.J. "Genetics for cardiologists" ReMedica Publ. London (UK), 2000

Figure 4.1 was from "Physiological Basis of Medical Practice" Brobeck J.R. Ed. Williams & Wilkins Co. Baltimore (USA), 1973

Figure 4.2 was from Bers D.M.: Cardiac excitation-contraction coupling. Nature 415: 198-205, 2002

Figure 4.3 was from Dumaine R. and Antzelevitch C.: Molecular Mechanisms underlying the Long-QT syndrome. Curr.Opin.Cardiol. 17: 36-42, 2002

I am indebted to the Authors for permission to use their figures as a source.

INDEX